Mass Casualty Incident Management in Germany
From Ramstein to Eschede

T Vemmer

MD FRCA DMCC

Dr T Vemmer, MD FRCA DMCC
Dept. of Anaesthetics
St George's Hospital
Blackshaw Road
London, SW17 0QT
DRTVEMMER@DOCTORSNET.CO.UK

Produced by:
Books on Demand GmbH
Gutenbergring 43
D-22848 Norderstedt
Germany

ISBN: 3 – 8334 – 0258 – X
This book can be obtained via www.amazon.de or www.libri.de

Pictures:
Most pictures copyright T Vemmer
Pictures in figures 2.7, 4.1, 7.1, 7.2, 7.3, and 7.4:
Grafik Team
Gusternhainer Straße 26b
D-35745 Herborn
Germany

Contents

List of Figures

List of Tables

Chapter 1

Abstract

The German emergency medical service is based on the cooperation of immediate care doctors and paramedics. For medical emergencies 'stay & stabilise' is the usual strategy, for trauma 'treat & run'. Training, equipment, and structures (e.g. helicopter emergency medical service) are presented.

The civil defence system is analysed in a historical context. Its evolution closely mirrors the changing concepts of war from the total war based on Clausewitz to van Creveld's low intensity conflicts of today: 'Transformation of war — transformation of civil defence'. It provides credible protection in the age of terrorism and small-scale warfare.

An audit tool for the assessment of the medical management of mass casualty incidents is developed based on the principles of total quality management. Checklists allow the audit of structural and process quality. The trimodal distribution of trauma death is found a useful tool for outcome assessment in both regular trauma systems and major incidents. The American paramedic system is shown to provide markedly inferior trauma care in comparison to the German physician-based system.

A case study of the aircrash at the Ramstein airshow 1988 highlights numerous problems with the traditional approach to incident management. Following a very open and public discussion of this event Germany improved the medical management of major incidents.

The three main areas of improvement were the command system

(DV100 incident management system allowing the integration of many different agencies and services, well trained medical and ambulance incident officers), the activation of reserves (mutual aid, rapid response teams, disaster control units, helicopter services, and military support), and the medical management (clear instructions for the first team on scene, clear structure of the incident site centered on the advanced medical post, triage, and dispersal to many trauma centres avoiding overload in one centre).

A case study on the high-speed train accident at Eschede 1998 shows the application of these principles in the real world. A final chapter considers the lessons which can be learned from the German changes.

Chapter 2

The Emergency Medical System

Emergency services are based on the idea of bringing the resuscitation room to the patient and not vice versa ('stay and stabilize' for medical emergencies, 'treat and run' for major trauma, figure 2.2, page 6). Outcomes show the German emergency medical system to be one of the best in the world, e.g. rates of neurologically intact survival after out of hospital cardiac arrest are higher than in many other countries[112]: Mainz 34%[237], Hamburg 33%[245], Göttingen 30%[27] In Seattle, USA, often seen as 'the golden standard' in the English-speaking world, only 12% leave the hospital (neurological outcome not given)[162].

The American trauma surgeon Trunkey considered the German trauma system and its outcomes exemplary[252].

In an emergency, bystanders are required by law to provide first aid and call the emergency services. Most citizens have participated in a first aid course, e.g. applicants for driving licences have to show proof of attendance, young men learn it during national service. In many jobs, e.g. heavy goods vehicle or bus drivers, an advanced first aid certificate is mandatory. Secondary schools often have first-aid groups run by pupils and teachers[129].

Ambulance control or a combined fire/ambulance control will receive all emergency calls and determine the level of response according to fixed protocols (predetermined attendance): ALS ambulance, prehospital emergency doctor, helicopter, or other services. Many controls will give telephone advice to encourage bystander

- unconcious patients, reduced level of consciousness

- severe or increasing dyspnoea

- respiratory arrest

- cardiac arrest

- (cardiac) chest pain

- shock/cardiovascular collapse of any cause

- severe haemorrhage

- major injuries, polytrauma

- entrapment

- suicide attempts

- intoxication/overdose

- obstetric emergencies

- seizures

- major incidents

- any requests by other doctors or qualified ambulance personnel

Table 2.1: Indication list for callout of prehospital emergency doctors

Note that all patients triaged 'red' in a British A&E department, and many people triaged 'yellow' will be seen by a prehospital emergency doctor at the scene.

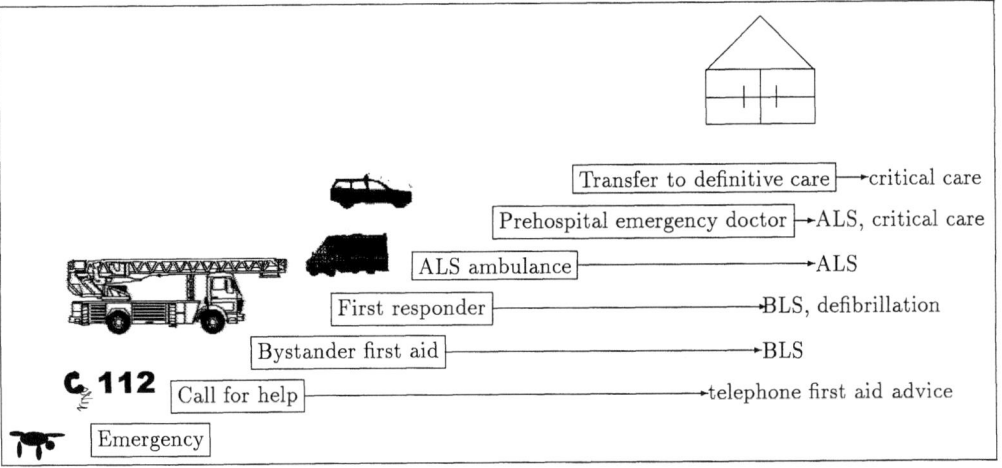

Figure 2.1: Chain of survival: Multi-tiered response to individual emergencies

first aid. More and more regions provide organized first responder schemes, e.g. by professional[93, 40] and volunteer fire brigades [77, 260] or aid associations[156, 164]. These first responders usually are well trained in basic life support with simple adjuncts and defibrillation. Public access defibrillaton projects are growing[233]. Professional fire brigades usually have their staff trained to paramedic or EMT-I (emergency medical technician – intermediate) level and fire engines are equipped to this standard[228]. The first responder will be followed by a paramedic ambulance, then the prehospital emergency physician's vehicle will arrive. Response times are set forth in state law, e.g. the mainly rural state of Lower Saxony requests maximum times of 8 minutes in urbanized and 12 minutes in rural areas, while the Hamburg fire brigade achieves response times of 5 minutes for paramedic and 8 minutes for the prehospital emergency physician ambulances [181].

Medical patients will usually be stabilized before transport ('stay and stabilize'), while the concept for trauma victims is 'treat and run'[22]. Patients with cardiac arrest are resuscitated on scene, and

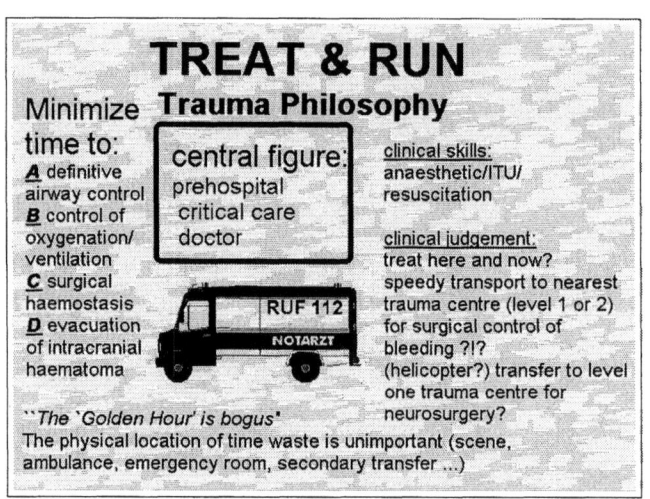

Figure 2.2: 'Treat and Run' trauma system

The prehospital emergency doctor not only got advanced skills, e.g. in airway management/emergency anaesthesia, the main task is the provision of clinical judgement on the scene. The time from trauma to definitive airway management and control of ventilation is minimised as in the French 'stay and stabilize' system, the time to surgical control of haemorrhage is at least as short as in the Anglo-American 'scoop and run'. The compromise, physician-led 'treat and run' is superior to systems run by protocol-based healthcare professionals, especially in neurotrauma (where 'scoop & run' to the next hospital causes long delays in the resuscitation room and on secondary transfers to a neurosurgical unit).

transported only after return of spontaneous circulation. CPR in an ambulance speeding to the next hospital is considered poor practice. If an arrest occurs during transport, the ambulance will stop to enable the driver/EMT-I to assist in the resuscitation. If not already on scene, an prehospital emergency doctor will be requested[86]. The patient will be transported to the next appropriate hospital, not the closest facility (trauma centres, available ITU beds, CT scanner, etc). Prior information of the hospital is the usual standard. The patient will be brought directly to the appropriate unit, e.g. ITU/CCU, medical admissions unit, shock room/theatre in case of major trauma... there are no long delays in an emergency department. Indeed, Germany does without the 'gatekeeper function' of Accident and Emergency Medicine, patients are seen directly by the appropriate specialty.

The states regulate the emergency services in their own jurisdiction without interference by the federal government. The responsibility for organizing and running fire and ambulance services rests with counties and cities. They may provide the ambulance service themselves, give the task to their fire brigade, or to third parties, e.g. aid associations or private providers. The four largest aid associations with their professional branches, German/Bavarian Red Cross (DRK/BRK)[1], Order of Malta Ambulance Service (MHD), Workers' Samaritans (ASB), and St John Ambulance (JUH) provide about 75% of ambulance services.

2.1 Personnel and Training

2.1.1 Notarzt — Prehospital Emergency Doctor

The immediate care/prehospital emergency doctor is at the centre of the emergency medical service. Minimum qualification for the prehospital emergency doctor is the certificate in prehospital medical care. It is awarded by the chamber of physicians after basic specialist training in an acute specialty, a minimum of 6 months

---

[1]The Free State of Bavaria got its own Red Cross association

experience in intensive care or anaesthetics, successful completion of an 80 hour course (incorporating ALS, PALS, trauma, etc.), and a number of supervised emergency callouts. These are minimum qualifications, the chambers of physicians of some states have further requirements, or offer higher qualifications, e.g. the chamber of physicians of the State of Lower Saxony awards a higher degree in prehospital emergency medicine. The base specialty of most prehospital emergency doctors is either anaesthetics or medicine, some come from trauma surgery or other specialties.

2.1.2 Paramedical Personnel

There are three levels of qualification for paramedical personnel: Rettungsassistent (≈ paramedic), Rettungssanitäter (≈ Emergency Medical Technician – intermediate, EMT-I) , and Rettungshelfer (≈ EMT-basic). Although most ambulances are staffed by professionals, there are some volunteers involved, especially in southern Germany. Volunteers must have the same formal qualifications as professional staff. Compulsory regular training (minimum 30h/ year of formal courses) helps to maintain standards.

Rettungsassistent — Paramedic

The Rettungsassistent (paramedic) is trained to provide skilled assistance to the prehospital emergency doctor and to treat patients independently, if required. Vocational training takes two years, with shorter courses for Rettungssanitäter (EMT-I), nurses, and non-commissioned officers of the armed forces medical service. Most professional fire brigades train their firefighters to paramedic standard. Often the general public not recognizing their high skill levels considers paramedics to be 'ambulance drivers'. Paramedics are skilled assistants in the prehospital environment, similar to operating department practitioners/anaesthetic nurses in the operating theatre or intensive care nurses in the ITU. Without skilled assistance critical care cannot be provided in ambulances, operating theatres, nor intensive care units. Prehospital emergency doctors and paramedics usually work in a symbiotic relationship of mutual professional respect. While on duty for doctor-manned vehicles, paramedics usually work in the base hospital, e.g. in ITU or the emergency department to maintain their high standard of training.

Rettungssanitäter — EMT-intermediate and Rettungshelfer — EMT-basic

Rettungssanitäter (EMT-I) have a minimum training of 520 hours (many courses are longer). They can work as drivers of ALS vehicles or team leaders on BLS ambulances. They are able to provide most advanced life support skills, e.g. intubation, defibrillation, i.v. access. Rettungshelfer (EMT-basic, EMT-B) have formal training of at least 160 hours. They serve as drivers of basic life support ambulances, can provide BLS and assist with advanced life support measures. Volunteers usually train to EMT-B level, some progress to EMT-I, few manage to become a Rettungsassistent (paramedic). First responders, e.g. volunteer firemen or members of aid organisations, are trained thoroughly in first aid and automated external defibrillation[121].

2.2 Equipment

Ambulances and equipment are normed (DIN 75080, part 1 – 3, German norm[2]). The types are Rettungswagen (RTW, ALS ambulance or mobile intensive care unit), Krankentransportwagen (KTW, BLS ambulance), Notarztwagen (NAW, prehospital emergency doctor ambulance/mobile intensive care unit), and Notarzteinsatzfahrzeug (NEF, prehospital emergency doctor speed intervention vehicle).

---

[2]The European norm (EN 1789) was not yet accepted during the study period. It is influenced heavily by the German norm

Specialist services like neonatal retrieval or ITU transfer teams are equipped with custom-made ground or air vehicles.

2.2.1 Rettungswagen RTW

Rettungstransportwagen (RTW), advanced life support/front line ambulances (figure 2.3, page 11) are used for patients in whom threatened vital functions have to be restored and maintained (DIN 75 080 part 1 and 2). The new European norm classifies these vehicles as type C ambulance (Mobile Intensive Care Unit). A large patient compartment with full standing height gives ample

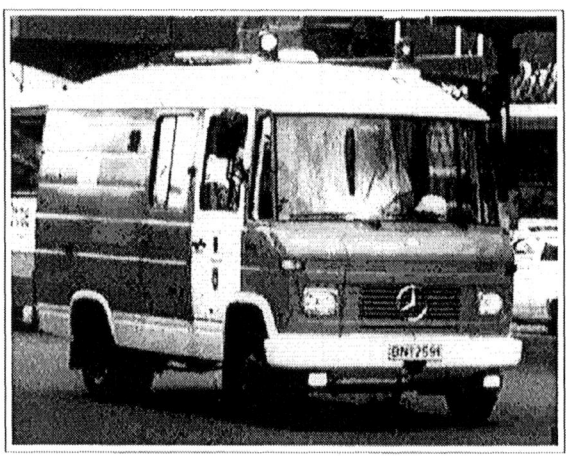

Figure 2.3: Rettungswagen RTW (advanced life support unit)

room for treatment. The stretcher is positioned in the middle of the vehicle, allowing access to the patient from three sides. The loading table for the stretcher can be elevated and brought into any position, e.g. Trendelenburg. The table got its own suspension to allow for a smooth ride. The vehicle is equipped to enable paramedics and doctors to deal with most emergency situations (table 2.2, page 11). Minimum staffing is one Rettungsassistent (paramedic) and one Rettungssanitäter (EMT-I). RTW are based on larger vans, often Volkswagen LT or Mercedes Benz vehicles.

defibrillator
oxygen delivery system (2 × 2200 l)
portable ventilator
intubation kit
portable and fixed suction units
crystalloid and colloid infusions with giving sets and cannulae
warming box for infusions
ample selection of drugs
emergency boxes/bags for airway/ventilation circulation paediatrics toxicology obstetrics
bags for replantates
vacuum mattress, orthopaedic scoop stretcher
splints
one stretcher, usually Stollenwerk or Ferno roll in type
many organisations use additional equipment not required by the norm, e.g. extra monitoring, depending on staff qualification

Normally, one patient only can be cared for at one time. Many providers of ambulance services equip their vehicles with one or more additional stretcher racks for use in major incidents only.

Table 2.2: Some of the equipment carried by Rettungswagen (RTW, advanced life support unit)

2.2.2   Krankentransportwagen KTW

Krankentransportwagen (KTW) or basic life support ambulances are normed (DIN 75 080 part 1 and 3, figure 2.4). These vehicles are mainly used for non-emergency work. Equipped to deal with emergencies until further help arrives (table 2.3, page 13), they may be used either as first responder units or in emergency situations where no RTWs (advanced life support units) are available. In major incidents they are commonly used to back up the front line services. Staffing is one Rettungssanitäter (EMT-intermediate) and one Rettungshelfer (EMT-basic). These are

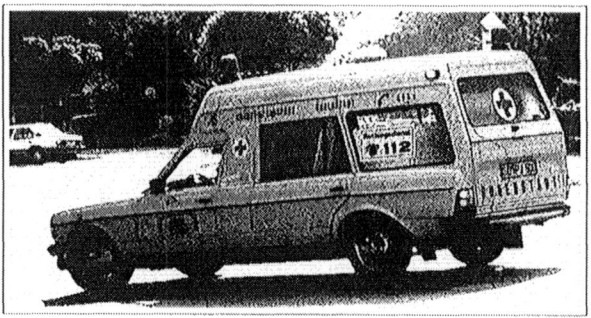

Figure 2.4: Krankentransportwagen KTW (basic life support unit)

minimum qualifications, often personnel with higher qualifications will be used. Like all emergency vehicles, the KTW will have blue flashlights and sirens. Most KTW are based either on small vans, market leader is the Volkswagen transporter, or on estates with an extended wheelbase and heightened roof. Compared to British ambulances, the KTW may be seen in the middle between patient transport vehicles and frontline units, probably coming closest to the ambulances used by the voluntary aid societies.

2.2.3 Notarztwagen NAW / Notarzteinsatzfahrzeug NEF — Prehospital Emergency Doctor's Vehicles

The idea behind the Notarztwagen (NAW, mobile intensive care unit) is to bring the resuscitation room, equipment, and team to the patient, instead of the patient to the resuscitation room at the hospital. It is a large RTW (advanced life support unit) with additional equipment for the prehospital emergency doctor, designed to provide a level of care at least equal to a hospital resuscitation room. Often these vehicles are adapted to the preferences of the respective senior emergency medical staff, but e.g. 12 lead ECG, a large choice of anaesthetic, cardiologic, and other drugs, central lines, a temporary pacemaker (external, but often also transoesophageal and transvenous), monitoring like capno-

oxygen delivery system (2 × 400 l)
self inflating ventilation bag
suction unit
crystalloid infusions (3 × 500 ml) with giving sets and cannulae
emergency obstetrical kit
first aid box
bags for replantates
nursing equipment
splints
orthopaedic scoop stretcher
vacuum mattress
two stretchers, one carrying chair
many organisations use additional equipment not required by the norm, e.g. defibrillator, ventilator, perfusor, drugs, intubation kit, etc., depending on staff qualification and intended use of the vehicle

Table 2.3: Some of the equipment carried by Krankentransportwagen (KTW, basic life support unit)

graphy, infusion pumps, advanced airway equipment, etc. can be expected. Many NAW carry more equipment, e.g. anaesthesia machine, burn kits ... A prehospital emergency doctor (Notarzt, NA), an experienced paramedic for skilled assistance and an EMT-intermediate driver form the team.

Alternatively, the NAW (mobile intensive care unit), the mobile resuscitation room, is formed by the meeting – 'rendez-vous' – of a RTW (advanced life support unit) and a Notarzteinsatzfahrzeug (NEF, immediate care doctor's car/speed intervention vehicle). This is a normal passenger car, often an estate or 4x4 (Volkswagen Passat Variant and Mercedes T models are the favourites), carrying all the mobile equipment of a NAW (emergency doctor ambulance) with the exception of the stretcher and the stationary equipment. It is staffed by a prehospital emergency doctor and either a para-medic or an EMT-intermediate as driver and skilled assistant[97].

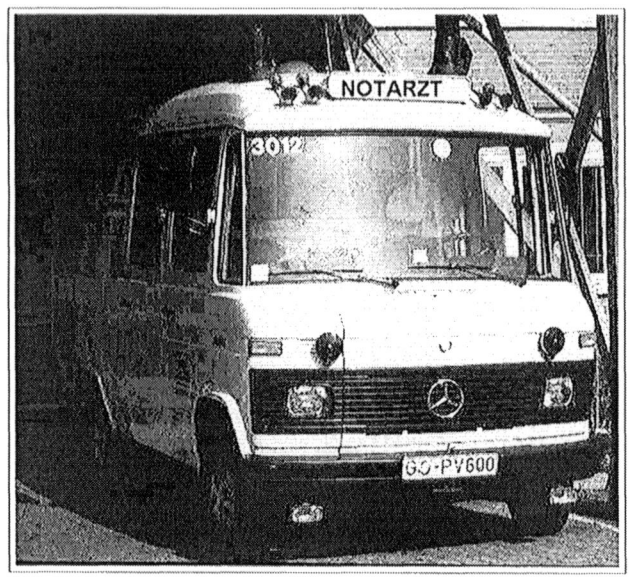

Figure 2.5: Notarztwagen — Mobile Intensive Care Unit

A fully equipped resuscitation room on wheels, staffed by an emergency doctor, a paramedic, and an EMT-I (driver).

2.2.4 Helicopter Services

56 emergency helicopter stations provide a comprehensive aero-medical system, covering the whole country in overlapping circles with a radius of 50km each. Providers are the federal minister of the interior (peacetime use of civil defence helicopters), the federal armed forces, an automobile club (ADAC), and two charities (DRF, Deutsche Rettungsflugwacht, and IFA, Internationale Flug Ambulanz). Emergency helicopters are staffed by a (senior) prehospital emergency doctor and an experienced flight paramedic, besides the pilot. The equipment is similar to the immediate care doctor vehicles. Common helicopter types are MBB Bo 105CBS, EC 135, Bell UH 1D, and BK117 with the capacity to transport one, in exceptional circumstances two patients. Helicopters are not used

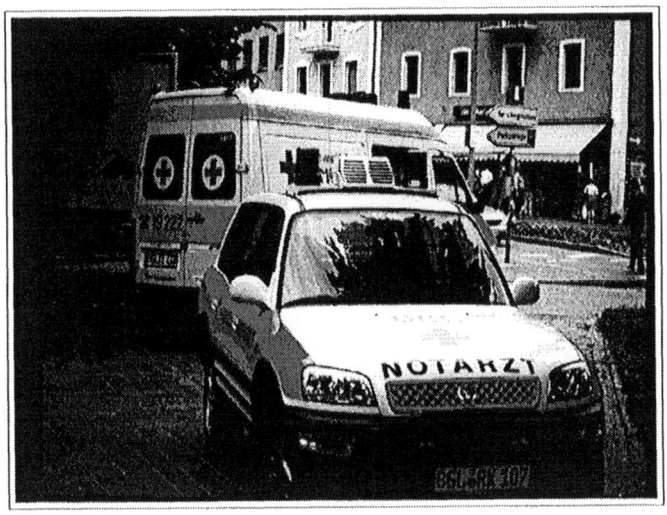

Figure 2.6: Notarzteinsatzfahrzeug, NEF, — Doctor's speed intervention car
Staffed by an emergency doctor and a paramedic driver. Always used
in conjunction with an ALS ambulance (RTW, background)

for 'scoop and swoop', but are fully integrated in the emergency
medical system. Tasks are:

- Rapid transport of doctor and paramedic to the scene

- provision of equal access to prehospital medical care for rural
  communities

- Immediate medical care and stabilisation

- Supporting the prehospital emergency doctor or ground ambulance crew already on scene (2nd on call function)

- Transport by ground ambulance of the stabilized patient ac-
  companied by doctor and flight paramedic

- Aeromedical evacuation from the scene to specialised (tertiary)
  care, e.g. neurosurgery, spinal injuries (primay transport)

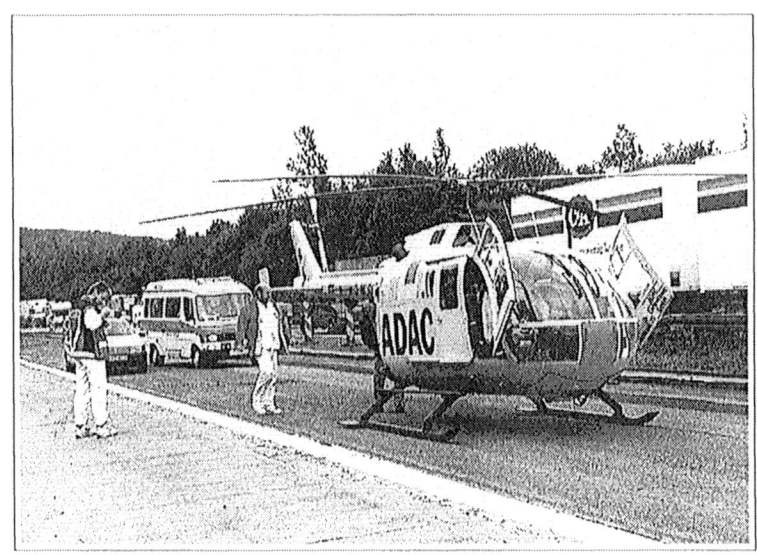

Figure 2.7: RTH — emergency helicopter

- Transport of emergency patients after stabilisation from small hospitals to tertiary centres (secondary transport)

- Transport of drugs, blood products, organs for transplantation, etc.

- Search and rescue of persons, e.g. in waterways or mountain areas

Cross-border cooperation is working well on a day to day basis, e.g. German helicopters and ground ambulances are saving patients in the border areas of Denmark, the Netherlands, Belgium, Luxembourg, France, Switzerland, and Austria, and vice versa[238]. Specialist intensive care transfer helicopters, usually with a larger patient compartment and extra equipment, e.g. Siemens Servo 300 ventilator, invasive monitoring, etc, provide a network for secondary transfers. They also serve as a backup to the normal emergency helicopters.

Chapter 3

Development of Civil Defence: From Clausewitz to van Creveld

This chapter describes the civil defence preparations in the Federal Republic of Germany (West Germany). Although the communist East German state had a rather well planned and equipped civil defence system, this was scrapped immediately after reunification, and structures along West German lines were put in place. The influence of the East German civil defence on major incident preparedness in the unified Germany was negligible.

3.1 Transformation of War — Transformation of Civil Defence

The evolution of civil defence in the Federal Republic of Germany closely mirrors the 'transformation of war' from the concept of 'total war' using maximal violence originally based on the thinking of Clausewitz to the low intensity conflicts of today[56, 66].

In the first years the aim was to protect the civilian population in a largely conventional war with some use of nuclear weapons between NATO and the Warsaw Pact, fought mainly in Germany. This was an extrapolation of the experiences gained in the second world war. In the classical teaching of Clausewitz, maximal violence would be used to achieve a political aim: World domination for the respective political system. Combatants would be clearly distinguished from non-combatants, the latter protected by the four Geneva conventions.

In the 1960s and 1970s a thermonuclear war leading to mutual destruction seemed a more likely scenario. The nuclear stalemate led to a reassessment of the role of civil defence. Britain dissolved its civil defence service in 1963. The German service was scaled down but never abandoned. After all, if anything had gone wrong, Germany would have been the battleground.

After the collapse of the Soviet empire and the reunification Germany found itself surrounded by friends and allies for the first time in history. The civil defence service underwent drastic reforms. Major incident and peacetime disaster management, a responsibility of the states, became far more important than preparing for a war unlikely to be fought in the foreseeable future. The only reason that the federal government did not completely abandon the provision of civil defence services was finance politics: The states, politically rather influential, were responsible for peacetime disaster preparedness, but either unwilling or unable to provide large investments in the emergency services. A compromise was reached: The states would organize emergency preparedness, funding would come out of both state and federal budgets.

An increasing threat of low intensity conflict/national and international terrorism[94] culminating in the attack on the World Trade Center (11th September 2001) forced a radical rethink: Germany, like most western societies, was a prime target in the era of low intensity conflict. In 1991 the Israeli military historian Martin van Creveld had described the 'transformation of war'[66]: Frequent, but localised attacks, mainly on the civilian population, potentially using weapons of mass effect, form a new scenario.

The aim of the attacker is no longer military victory (or mutual annihilation), but intimidation of the population, influencing public opinion. Main task of the government must be to fortify the attitudes of the population. Being prepared, the ability to provide efficient aid after a terrorist attack, is an important part of defending democracy against this threat.

The effects of terrorist attacks would be similar to those of major accidents. Civil defence and the normal emergency services need to be integrated closely. The changes implemented after the re-unification proved to be a blessing in disguise: The integrated structures were already there, all what was needed were some additional resources. The message both at home and abroad is clear: Germany is prepared for low intensity conflict[24, 150].

3.2 Luftschutzhilfsdienst — Air Raid Protection Service

After the second world war Germany was governed by the victors who did not permit suspicious 'paramilitary' activities like disaster or civil emergency preparedness. The main problem was the running of a humble everyday ambulance and fire service anyway.

The constitution of the newly founded Federal Republic of Germany (West Germany, 1949) divided the responsibilty for emergency management between the different levels of government. People had enough of being told what to do by central government 'leaders'. Under the new constitution, decisions would be taken as close to the people as possible, at the lowest level of government. For the emergency services this meant that the federal government stayed responsible for (wartime) civil defence, the states provided (peacetime) disaster management and had the right to legislate emergency planning, while local county or city councils were running fire, ambulance, and other emergency services.

To join the NATO, the new Federal Republic of Germany had to reestablish a national defence system, comprising both armed forces and protection of the civilian population. The federal ministry of the interior ($\approx$ home office) was made responsible for civil defence.

The new system was modelled on the second world war air raid

Command Section	command car 3 motorbikes	CL/D PL R Dr/R 3MC	2/0/5
1st Medical Platoon			1/9/20
Command Squad	car	PL/D R Dr	1/0/2
1st Section	12 stretcher ambulance	SL SqL SqL Dr 5M	0/3/6
2nd Section	12 stretcher ambulance	SL SqL SqL Dr 5M	0/3/6
3rd Section	12 stretcher ambulance	SL SqL SqL Dr 5M	0/3/6
2nd Medical Platoon			1/9/20
	As 1st Platoon		
3rd Medical Platoon			1/9/20
	As 1st Platoon		
Support Platoon			1/1/9
Command Squad	van motorbike	PL Dr M MC	1/0/3
Kitchen	lorry/field kitchen	SL/Pr Dr C	0/1/6
Support	lorry/generator 5KVA	Dr M	
Ambulance	3 stretcher ambulance	Dr M	
total	111 stretcher cases		6/28/74

Figure 3.1: Mobile Medical Company (1965)

The vehicles marked with an asterisk were to be requisitioned from private owners. CL = Company Leader, PL = Platoon Leader, SL = Section Leader, SqL = Squad Leader, D = Doctor, C = Cook, Pr = Purser, Dr = Driver, MC = Motorcycle Courier, R = Radio Operator, M = Man. Rightmost column: Numbers of officers/non-commissioned officers/men protection service which had shown its efficiency during the 'thousand bomber' raids. A well organized aid system had been able to cope even with the big city fire storms[107].

An updated version of this had to be able to alleviate the effects of an atomic war.

Large, autonomous, motorized units were the centrepiece of the new Luftschutzhilfsdienst (LSHD, air raid protection service), able to provide assistance over large distances — only the support from other areas had enabled the emergency services of the fire storm cities to deal with an attack which otherwise must have overwhelmed even the best efforts.

Self help of the affected population was considered crucial (e. g. fireguards, first aid). The federal government sponsored free first aid training for the general public and free training courses for auxiliary nurses (for auxiliary and military hospitals)[194].

The LSHD was divided into specialty services:

Communications

Fire

Rescue

Medical

NBC

Welfare

Warning

Veterinary

Repair of public utilities

Support

These services complemented the 'self protection' of the citizens. The medical service had sheltered and unprotected auxiliary hospitals, first aid posts, mobile medical companies, local (motorized) medical companies, and motorized patient transport platoons[102]. Doctors, other officers, and specialists trained at the federal civil defence training centre, non-commissioned officers at regional schools, and men were trained locally in advanced first aid, basic

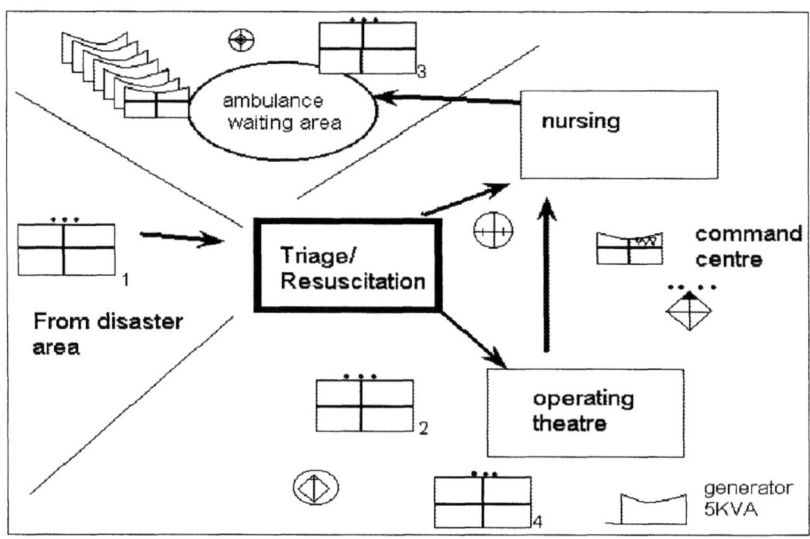

Figure 3.2: Civil Defence dressing station, 1965 regulations

The mobile medical company provided a 'Schwerpunkt' in such a
dressing station which could be either in suitable buildings or in
tents[42]. The first medical platoon (1) provided help in the disaster
area and transported the injured to the dressing station. The
second medical platoon (2), with the support platoon (4), ran the
dressing station, while the third medical platoon (3) was in charge of
ambulance transport. The arrows indicate patient flow.

ambulance care, and protection against nuclear, biological, and chemical weapons.

The mobile medical companies were intended to provide a 'Schwerpunkt'[1] (see box) at the site of a major incident.

> **Schwerpunkt** ('focal point') — Concept created by Carl von Clausewitz[56]. (Military) resources should not be spread out thinly, but concentrated in one main thrust to achieve local superiority. The idea proved successful not only in war (e.g.'Blitzkrieg'), but also in business, politics, and other fields.

The company consisted of a command section with a 4x4 radio command car and motorcycle couriers, three medical platoons equipped with three large capacity ambulances each (12 stretchers, four wheel drive), and a support platoon with an ambulance (3 stretchers, for the severely wounded)[134], a van, and two lorries (figure 3.1, page 20)[188].

The sturdy 12 stretcher four wheel drive ambulances came in useful during the flood disaster in Hamburg 1962 and during the snow catastrophe in Lower Saxony 1978. Constructed like military vehicles, they were not normally considered fit for peacetime use[97]. The local medical companies were structured similarly. Each 12 stretcher ambulance was replaced by two tilted lorries carrying easily mounted racks for six stretchers each (Krankenlastkraftwagen, KrLKW, auxiliary lorry ambulance). While the federal civil defence administration provided the equipment, the command car, the ambulances, and the stretcher racks, the lorries, motorcycles, and vans had to be requisitioned from private owners, feasible only in wartime.

The mobile medical company had the task to:

---

[1]I have not found a good English translation for this concept, even British historians use the German expression[30, 88]

23

Command Squad	radio van motorcycle	PL CSqL Dr MC	1/1/2
Medical Section	ambulance (4) ambulance (8)	2D SL SqL 4M 2Dr	2/2/6
1st First Aid Section	ambulance (4) ambulance (4)	SL SqL 8M 2Dr	0/2/10
2nd First Aid Section	ambulance (4) ambulance (4)	SL SqL 8M 2Dr	0/2/10
3rd First Aid Section	ambulance (4) ambulance (4)	SL SqL 8M 2Dr	0/2/10
total	36 stretcher cases		3/9/38

Figure 3.3: Structure of the medical platoon (1976 reforms)

397 such platoons covered all areas of West Germany.
The vehicles marked with an asterisk were to be requisitioned from
private owners. Ambulance (4) = 4 stretchers, ambulance (8) =
8 stretchers. The 4 stretcher ambulance of the medical section
was equipped for advanced, the others for basic life support. D
= Doctor, PL= Platoon Leader, CSqL = Command Squad Leader
(deputy platoon leader), SL = Section Leader, SqL = Squad Leader,
Dr = Driver, MC = Motorcycle Courier, M = Man

- set up a dressing station either in existing buildings or in tents

- accept the injured rescued by the fire or rescue services

- support the fire or rescue service on scene (e.g. entrapped
  casualties)

- cooperate with the NBC service in the decontamination of
  casualties exposed to non-conventional weapons

- register all casualties

- triage

- stabilize patients using basic and advanced life support

- provide life-saving interventions in a field operating theatre

- hold patients in a nursing area

- allocate patients to receiving hospitals

- transport patients to regular and auxiliary hospitals

- support other units of the medical service (medical platoons, first aid posts, regular and auxiliary hospitals) as required

The dressing station was structured into areas for receiving casualties (registration, triage), resuscitation, emergency theatre, nursing, and ambulance waiting and loading areas (figure 3.2, page 22).

The companies were staffed by volunteers and conscripts. As volunteers were not coming forward in large enough numbers, the units were handed over to the aid organisations. Red Cross, Order of Malta, Workers' Samaritans, and St John Ambulance would provide the volunteers and would in exchange be allowed to use vehicles and equipment for their own purposes. A positive side effect was increased training and experience of the helpers, e.g. at mass gatherings or sport events.

3.3 Erweiterter Katastrophenschutz/Zivilschutz — Enhanced Disaster Protection/Civil Protection

In 1968 political pressure lead to a reform of the LSHD. The name was changed to 'erweiterter Katastrophenschutz/Zivilschutz' (KatS/ZS, 'enhanced' disaster protection/civil protection, the 'enhancement' being a polite expression for the now no longer politically correct war time air raid protection).

In 1976 the companies were dissolved, as they had been far too unwieldy for any peacetime use and replaced by smaller, more flexible platoons.

The medical service now had three types of platoons: dressing station, medical, and ambulance/patient transport. Basic Ford

Command Squad	radio van motorcycle	PL CSqL Dr MC	1/1/2
Medical Section	2 squad vehicles lorry ambulance	2D SL 2SqL 3Dr 6M	2/3/9
1st First Aid Section	first aid section van	SL SqL Dr 5M	0/2/6
2nd First Aid Section	first aid section van	SL SqL Dr 5M	0/2/6
3rd First Aid Section	first aid section van	SL SqL Dr 5M	0/2/6
Ambulance Section	ambulances (4 stretchers)	SL SqL 4Dr 2M	0/2/6
total	36 stretcher cases		3/12/35

Figure 3.4: Medical platoon, 1984

485 platoons were strategically distributed all over Germany[43]. The vehicles marked with an asterisk were to be requisitioned from private owners. Auxiliary ambulances: The medical squad vehicles could be converted to 4 stretcher ambulances, the lorry ambulance carried six stretchers in three stretcher racks, and the first aid section vans had two stretchers each. Abbreviations as in figure 3.3, page 24

Transit four stretcher ambulances (nicknamed 'federal wheelbarrows' by the civil defence medics)[48] became the workhorse of the service (Figure 3.3, page 24)[194]. The large capacity 12 stretcher ambulances were converted to 8 stretcher ambulances. The middle row of stretchers was removed to allow access to the patients for some basic care.

In the meantime, the old 'scoop and run' ambulance service had evolved into an emergency medical service with immediate care doctors, trained ambulance personnel, advanced life support vehicles, etc. This was not reflected in civil defence planning, the units were still nothing more than dumbed down economical versions of their second world war counterparts.

Training and exercises still prepared for the defence situation, cooperation with normal emergency services was not considered to be important. On the other hand, the peacetime emergency medical services with the focus on individual patients had not much use for their poorly trained and equipped civil defence counterparts.

They were rarely used in real emergencies.

The 1980s saw an overhaul of the medical platoons. The old vehicles of the 1950s and 1960s were worn out by now and needed replacing, a war seemed more unlikely than ever, and prehospital emergency medicine had made such progress that it appeared to be worlds apart from civil defence medical care. In the medical platoon the large capacity ambulance was replaced by two Arzttruppkraftwagen (ATrKw, medical squad vehicle), carrying personnel and more modern equipment.

Ford Transit 4 stretcher ambulances[49] and Sanitätsgruppenkraftwagen (SanGrKw, first aid section van)[52, 53] provided transport for the other elements of the unit (figure 3.4, page 26).

The dressing station and the ambulance platoons were changed to medical platoon (doctor) and medical platoon (transport) respectively. All three different medical platoons now had the same task despite different equipment and personnel, creating a 'Schwerpunkt' at major incident sites, triaging, stabilising, and transporting patients. This allowed Civil Defence administrators to claim there where enough medical platoons for all possible emergencies, even though many (medical platoon (doctor) and medical platoon (transport) — the latter did not even have doctors — were just incomplete versions of the medical platoon.

The Arzttruppkraftwagen (medical squad vehicle) was a large Mercedes-Benz van, staffed by a doctor, a non-commissioned officer, three men, and a driver. In the back it carried four stretchers for use as an auxiliary ambulance. Using the vehicle as an ambulance was not normally permitted in times of peace. It was equipped with a tent and materials for setting up a small field dressing station[46, 47]. These vehicles are still widely used today.

The helpers were alerted either by siren signals or by telephone snowballing. Most platoons were ready for deployment several hours after the initial alert only, while requisitioning of private vehicles would have taken days and would have been unrealistic in peacetime incidents. Real alerts were considered to be very unlikely indeed.

There was one shining exception to this rather bleak scene: The federal civil defence administration allowed the use of its helicopters for peacetime emergency work. Intended for command, control, and reconnaissance in the aftermath of a thermonuclear attack, the helicopters were stationed at trauma centres, equipped to the full German norm for air ambulances, and staffed by experienced pre-hospital emergency doctors and flight paramedics. 16 of the 56 emergency helicopter stations are using a total of 24 civil defence helicopters[54, 123].

3.4 Civil Defence after the End of the Cold War

The reunification of Germany brought the end of Civil Defence as it had existed up to then. For the first time in history, Germany was surrounded by friends and allies only. Why waste money on defence any more? Even the federal armed forces suffered marked cuts in their budget and had to prove their right to continuing existence in UN/NATO peacekeeping missions. Huge economic discrepancies between Western Germany and the east run down by over forty years of communist dictatorship had to be addressed by a large reconstruction programme. The federal budget became very tight suddenly.

The result for Civil Defence was predictable: The federal govern-

Command Squad	radio van	PL CSqL Dr 2M	1/1/3
1st Medical Section Medical Squad	squad vehicle	D SL Dr 2M	1/1/3
Ambulance Squad	ambulance (4 stretchers)	SqL Dr 2M	0/1/3
2nd Medical Section	as 1st section		1/2/6
3rd Medical Section	as 1st section		1/2/6
4th Medical Section	as 1st section		1/2/6
total	32 stretcher cases		5/9/36

Figure 3.5: Medical platoon, Free State of Bavaria

This is essentially an improved version of the federal civil defence unit. All vehicles are immediately available, no time consuming requisitioning of private vehicles. Four doctors and more equipment make this platoon a useful support for peacetime emergency medical services. Each medical section can be called separately as a rapid response team, e.g. to smaller incidents. All volunteers carry pagers for a fast alert. Abbreviations as in figure 3.3, page 24

ment tried to reduce its obligations as much as possible. Now the Ministry of the Interior would no longer provide a full scale civil defence system. Only core services were retained (fire, medical, rescue, welfare, NBC). The platoons were dissolved, instead the states were given 'equipment kits'[41].

The medical service equipment kit consisted of two Arzttrupp-kraftwagen (medical squad vehicle — by now cheaper Fiat instead of Mercedes Benz) and four four-stretcher ambulances (first Ford Transit[50], then Mercedes obtained the tender with its Sprinter vans[51, 196]). The number of equipment kits related to the population of the state[7].

The federal government paid for the additional training of the helpers for wartime only. The units of the states, strengthened by the federal equipment kits, have to deal with both peacetime disasters and the defence situation (federal civil defence act 1997)

[269, 239]. The states were allowed to distribute the vehicles of the equipment kits as they saw fit and to integrate the civil defence helpers into state units.

Most states had simply relied on the federal civil defence units for peacetime major incident work. After all, the number of volunteers was limited, and public money could be spent in other areas more attractive to tax payers.

Sponsoring large fire departments to buy bus ambulances and medical equipment container pods for existing prime movers was seen as more cost effective: The equipment was fully integrated into normal emergency services and running costs would be paid by the respective borough or county, not the state[163, 159].

Some states, e.g. Hessia and North-Rhine Westphalia provided peacetime disaster services at state level, including medical units of platoon strength[143, 103].

This was often determined by political expediency. In the wake after the Ramstein air show incident, Baden-Württemberg, the richest state, even bought its own medical squad vehicles (Arzttruppkraftwagen). Unlike its counterpart of the federal civil defence it was fully equipped to advanced life support ambulance standard, a genuinely useful vehicle for peacetime major incidents [31].

The state of Lower Saxony had recurrent problems with brush and woodland fires. Most of its major incident budget went into the provision of 4x4 forest fire appliances for volunteer fire brigades. For the medical management of major incidents Hanover relied on the federal civil defence provisions.

The usefulness of these state disaster units was limited. Instead of two parallel systems, peacetime emergency services and federal civil defence, there were three parallel systems which met and cooperated on rare occasions, mainly at large scale exercises. Not infrequently helpers were members of more than one level of response, e.g. working in a professional ambulance service and volunteering in a civil defence medical platoon[35, 34].

The paradigm shift in major incident planning at the end of the 1980s and the consequences to the civil defence system of the political upheaval after the reunification (not only did the Russians not invade the West, they even left the East of Germany, taking away much of the legitimation for civil defence) forced the states to rethink their disaster planning.

Civil defence helpers were trained and available, all they needed was a worthwile task[104].

Rapid response teams of volunteers and off-duty professional medical and ambulance personnel seemed to sprout out of the earth everywhere.

The new principle of incident management was a timely support of the normal emergency medical service by the rapid response teams, followed by state disaster control units[241].

The main problem of the rapid response teams was a lack of standardisation[110]. A rapid response team can comprise anything from a small group of volunteers in a Volkswagen van[222] to large units of off-duty emergency doctors and paramedics with mobile intensive care units and ALS ambulances[161, 84], some are even equipped to deal with chemical incidents[96, 225].

Clearly, some regulation and standardisation was needed.

The first wave of states to deal with this problem came up with a number of different solutions:

Bavaria created an improved medical platoon (figure 3.5, page 29)[36].

Brandenburg came up with a new unit: Rapid Medical Response Team (Brandenburg), with vehicles to state specification (figure 3.6, page 32)[58, 57, 59]. This unit is designed to integrate with the normal emergency medical services.

Its welfare service mutated to a psychosocial crisis intervention team, seven helpers in a Ford Transit van, trained to provide critical incident stress debriefing and counselling to the affected population and the aid teams[113].

North-Rhine Westphalia found that its state medical platoons were

Triage & Treatment			
1st Team	response van	TL D 5EMT-I	2/0/5
2nd Team	response van	DTL D 5EMT-I	1/1/5
Technical Team	technical van	TTL Dr 2M	0/1/3
total	no transport		3/2/13

Figure 3.6: Rapid medical response team, State of Brandenburg

Each triage and treatment team is equipped to treat 20 patients. Equipment and qualifications of the team members is to normal civilian standards. The unit does not transport patients. It provides a casualty treatment station or works at the incident site. Abbreviations as in figure 3.3, page 24. TL = Team Leader, DTL = Deputy Team Leader, EMT-I = Emergency Medical Technician — Intermediate, TTL = Technical Team Leader

as inflexible and impractical as the federal civil defence units. They trialled a downsized light medical platoon, without doctor or advanced equipment (figure 3.7, page 33)[168]. It had a purely supportive role at major incidents, dealing with minor injuries, walking wounded, and noninjured persons. This was a new concept, all other states kept the main task of their major incident units the structuring of the scene and the provision of a casualty treatment station. North-Rhine Westphalia soon returned to a more conventional model.

The German Red Cross came up with the concept of the 'Emergency Unit', consisting of a command squad, a medical, a welfare, and a technical support section (figure 3.8)[169]. Subsequently most states implemented variations of the Red Cross concept as their major incident units[11].

The close integration of state disaster protection and federal civil defence proved ideal for the changing times: Low intensity conflict dominates the agenda of emergency planning[218].

Command Squad	command van motorcycle	PL CSqL Dr MC	1/1/2
1st Section	aux. ambulance	SL SqL Dr 5M	0/2/6
2nd Section	aux. ambulance	SL SqL Dr 5M	0/2/6
Technical Squad	van	SqL Dr M	0/1/2
total	4 stretcher cases		1/6/16

Figure 3.7: Medical platoon, trial version, State of North-Rhine Westphalia
Without doctor, without any advanced life support capability, able to transport four minor stretcher cases only, the tactical value of this platoon was low. The main task would have been to take care of the walking wounded and the uninjured. North-Rhine Westphalia soon replaced it with units based on the German Red Cross model (figure 3.8, page 34). Abbreviations: See figure 3.3, page 24. Aux. ambulance = auxiliary ambulance, a van carrying two stretchers

Scenarios become interchangeable between peacetime accidents and terrorist attacks: Trains derail because of human and technical errors or because of sabotage, buses and coaches crash or fall prey to suicide bombers, violence in organized crime and terrorism is often similar, accidents involving hazardous materials require a similar response to weapons of mass effect [210] ...

The training course for civil defence doctors at the federal civil defence training centre in Bad Neuenahr–Ahrweiler now incorporates the syllabus recommended by the International Society for Disaster Medicine[2].

The federal government stepped up its support for civil defence, currently focussing on the provision of 4 stretcher ambulances[51] and NBC reconnaissance vehicles — the soft skin civil defence equivalent of the Spürfuchs (fox) armoured NBC detector/analyser unit[45], all to be integrated into the state run disaster preparedness programs.

Through a slow process of modernisation the civil defence system

Command Squad	command van	PL CSqL Dr	1/1/1
Medical Section	squad vehicle ambulance (4 stretchers)	D SL 8M	1/1/8
Welfare Section			
Social Care Squad	van	SL Dr 2M	0/1/3
Accommodation Squad	van	SqL Dr 2M	0/1/3
Feeding Squad	lorry/field kitchen	SqL C Dr 2M	0/1/4
Technical Squad	van	SqL Dr 2M	0/1/3
total	12 stretcher cases		2/6/22

Figure 3.8: Emergency Unit, model proposed by the German Red Cross

Most states base their state disaster units on this model. The command squad and the medical section together form a rapid response team. The unit is equipped to support the regular emergency medical service (advanced first aid for 20 patients) and to provide welfare aid for up to 500 persons. The technical squad gives the unit a degree of autonomy (shelter, water, floodlights, electricity, ...) Abbreviations as in figures 3.1, page 20 and 3.3, page 24

is changing to meet the needs of today. The times when civil defence equalled air raid protection are gone. The modern enemy does no longer flatten the cities in thousand bomber raids or a thermonuclear apocalypse. The enemies of today work from within, blowing up buses as suicide bombers, distributing sarin in underground stations, anthrax spores in the mail, attacking government buildings, and terrorising the population.

A modern civil defence system must be capable of dealing with such threats. The German civil defence provides credible protection in today's era of low intensity conflict.

Chapter 4

An Audit Tool for the Medical Management of Major Incidents

In the decade between 1988 and 1998 the medical management of major incidents changed fundamentally. Did these changes result in an improved outcome for patients? There is no simple measurement to assess the quality of incident management. In this chapter I will develop an audit tool to do so. The aim is to evaluate the response of the emergency medical service to the disasters described in the case studies (Ramstein and Eschede) and to compare it to the response to similar incidents elsewhere. Total quality management comprises structural, process, and outcome quality. Applied to disaster medicine, structural and process quality are relatively easy to assess: Structural quality are the resources available, process quality evaluates how an incident was handled, e.g. compliance with guidelines. Outcome quality is more difficult to measure. Unlike structure and process quality, outcomes can easily be compared between different emergency medical systems. The main focus of this chapter will be the use of the trimodal distribution of trauma death as an outcome indicator in mass casualty incidents.

4.1 Structural and Process Quality

Auditing structures and processes is easy, once standards are established to audit against. Unfortunately, while many – often incompatible – standards have been set, little or no international agreement exists about even the most basic requirements and procedures. Good examples are 'triage' and 'dispersal'. While 'triage' is an accepted procedure since the Napoleonic wars, even inside a single country like Germany there still are incompatible triage systems and categories[190]. 'Dispersal' means the distribution of patients to a number of different hospitals in order to avoid overwhelming one hospital and to provide individual treatment as soon as possible. Introduced by Nicolai Ivanovich Pirogov during the Crimean war and widely adopted in continental Europe[215], the principle of 'dispersal' is only just reaching the English-speaking countries. The Advanced Life Support Group in their 2002 edition of the 'Major Incident Medical Management and Support' student manual[119] does not even mention it.

For an audit of the medical management of mass casualty incidents in Germany, it seems reasonable to identify standards accepted in Germany, even if they may be applied to other countries with difficulty only. The main purpose is to evaluate the management of the two incidents described in the case studies. The three chapters between the case studies deal mainly with improvements in structural and process quality. Two tables summarize useful standards for audit (tables 4.1 and 4.2, pages 37, 38).

4.2 Outcome Quality

Indicators of outcome are often arbitrary: Mortality, morbidity, survivors, scores, or even the time until the site of the incident has been cleared of patients. Trauma scoring systems, e.g. NACA, TRISS, RTS, or burns scores (Koblenz, body surface area,...) are aimed at individual patients. Subsequently they can be related to

standards and measures	source
Regular emergency services:	
Availability of emergency doctors, helicopters	178
ALS, and BLS ambulances within 15, 30, and 60 min	
(radius of 10, 20, and 40 km (ground) or 50, 100, and 200 km(air))	
rapid response teams within 20/40 km	36
state disaster units/ civil defence within 20/40 km	36
military/ other support within 60 min	146
standard: 1 doctor for 5 patients	201
standard: 1 'helper' (from paramedic to civil defence	201
aidman) for 1 patient	
qualification of aid personnel	209
medical command structure:	
medical incident officer	189
ambulance incident officer	189
command support	203
advanced medical post: team and equipment	208
trauma centers (level 1 – 3) within a distance of	200
30/60 minutes by ground/ by air	
burns beds within 60 minutes	105

Table 4.1: Audit standards of structural quality

mortality or other outcome measures. The main problem is the use of many different systems making it impossible to compare the outcomes in different major incidents. Inflexible, protocol-driven triage systems, e.g. 'Simple Triage And Rapid Treatment' (START) or its British adaptation, the 'triage sieve', will always put patients in the same triage category, irrespective of the actual number of casualties. Such systems could form the basis of a useful audit tool, relating triage categories to mortality or another outcome measure. While intuitively appealing, this approach is not feasible:

— START/'triage sieve' results are documented rarely in case reports of major incidents. They are nearly never correlated to mortality.

— Burns patients tend to be undertriaged by this system. Often patients with major burns are able to walk initially and are triaged as T3/'green' walking wounded, even though their injuries may be

standards and measures	source
first team does not start treatment	255
provides short feedback to control	255
gains an overview	255
establishes command & control	255
first command: "transport stop" — no spontaneous, uncontrolled transports to hospitals	255
reserves: time for control to mobilize backup were mutual aid, rapid response teams, disaster units, civil defence, the military, and independent providers called early? not enough or too many reserves mobilized?	204
triage use of established categories initial, e.g. START flexible, adapted to situation or protocol-based? dynamic, repeated over-/undertriage	64 256
stabilisation of 'immediate' patients before transport	100
inappropriate procedures, e.g. CPR	262
handover to medical/ ambulance incident officers	255
communication sufficient, breakdown of radio network?	117
advanced medical post established	208
ambulance waiting area	186
no self-deployment of ambulances/ teams ('disaster tourism')	
dispersal to different hospitals	105, 257
number of secondary (hospital to hospital) transfers	

Table 4.2: Audit standards of process quality

unsurvivable. The first case study describes the Ramstein airshow incident with its numerous burns patients. An audit tool based on START/'triage sieve' will not give a fair measurement in such an incident.
— START/'triage sieve' are often used in emergency systems without or with only very limited medical input. Such systems are not often applied in European physician-led trauma systems. For major incidents in Germany START/'triage sieve' does not form a useful audit tool, because it is not used frequently.
The trimodal distribution of trauma death [252] can be used as a

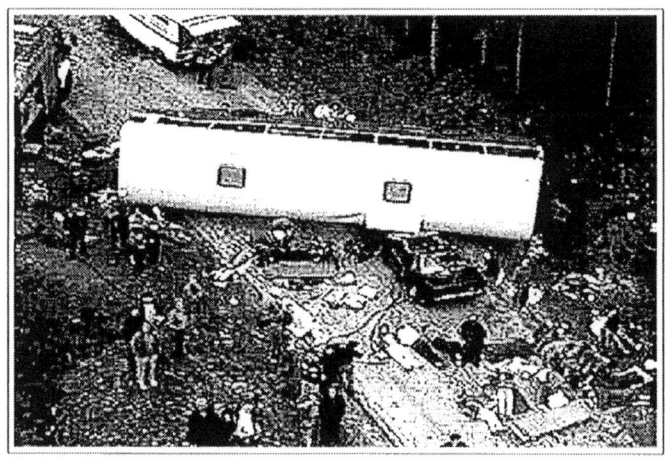

Figure 4.1: Coach accident

year	dead	1st	2nd	3rd	injured	source
2001	3	2	1	0	28	135
2000	6	5	1	0	22	12
1999	2	1	0	1	26	32
1999	3	1	2	0	40	259
1999	2	1	1	0	27	216
1999	1	0	0	1	17	165
1998	3	3	0	0	49	133
1997	4	2	2	0	7	131
1997	2	2	0	0	29	266
1996	7	7	0	0	26	170
1996	1	1	0	0	38	4
1994	8	6	0	2	40	191
1994	4	4	0	0	13	236
1992	20	19	1	0	31	234

Table 4.3: Ten years of coach accidents in Germany

Dead = total sum of fatalities; 1st, 2nd, and 3rd refer to the modes of the trimodal distribution of trauma deaths; injured = injured survivors realistic audit tool. It is based on a 'proper body count', data is often available easily, or can be put together retrospectively. It is a 'quick and dirty' approach which can be applied anywhere, to any trauma system. The necessary data can often be abstracted from reports of major incidents. The three modes reflect on the quality of care available: The first mode, immediate deaths, happen independently of the trauma care provided, the second (early deaths) reflect on the trauma system, while the third mode, late deaths, occur subsequently in hospital. A good trauma system should have a fairly low proportion of (early) deaths in the second mode and of late deaths. To form a baseline, the average of many incidents is taken — each individual incident may have been particularly fortunate or unfortunate, the average shows a general trend.

4.3 Trimodal Distribution of Trauma Death

In 1983 Donald D Trunkey first described the trimodal distribution of trauma deaths[252]: 50% of trauma fatalities happen immediately, within seconds to minutes of the impact. Common causes of death are massive damages to major vessels or severe head injuries. These patients are killed before any medical intervention can take place, their number can be reduced by prevention, e.g. use of seatbelts, only. The second mode ($\approx 30\%$) occurs minutes to hours after the accident. Fatalities are caused by obstruction of airways, breathing difficulties, and massive haemorrhage, usually caused by severe head or torso injuries. In these patients emergency medical systems can make a huge difference. The third mode of late deaths ($\approx 20\%$) in the days and weeks after the trauma is mainly due to complications of critical care, e.g. multi-organ failure, infections/sepsis, or pulmonary embolism. Emergency medical care can decrease such complications. Trauma surgeons from Munich were able to show a marked reduction in the incidence of multi-organ failure and mortality after early intubation and ventilation[253].

4.3.1 Baseline Data

Trunkey's original numbers[252], the outcomes of an American paramedic system (Denver, Colorado)[221], and those of recent coach accidents in Germany form a baseline for comparison. Coach accidents were chosen because they represent major incidents of a limited scale (figure 4.1, page 39).

Methods

German prehospital emergency care journals were hand searched for case reports of coach accidents. Inclusion criteria were:
Coach accident
Multiple casualties: $\geq$ 10 casualties
Severity: Impact severe enough to cause mortality
Survivability: At least one casualty survives the impact
Clear account of incident published
Location: Incident took place in Germany
Time frame: Decade between 1992 and 2001
I limited myself to the decade between 1992 and 2001 to assess recent accidents in which presumably care of a decent quality (to the standards accepted in Germany) had been provided. 14 case reports were sufficiently detailed (table 4.3, page 39). The three data sets used as baseline differed widely (figure 4.2, page 42). Half of Trunkey's fatalities occured immediately after the accident. The German coach accident trauma deaths peaked even more in the immediate period, while the Denver trauma system had the highest mortality in the second mode (minutes to hours). A modern trauma system could be expected to provide better outcomes than the American system of the late 1970s and early 1980s. Trunkey described a trauma system at its inception. Advanced Trauma Life Support (ATLS) was adopted by the American College of Surgeons in 1980 [60], probably most of Trunkey's patients did not yet profit from its standardized approach. Prehospital care was mostly limited to a simple 'scoop & run' approach.

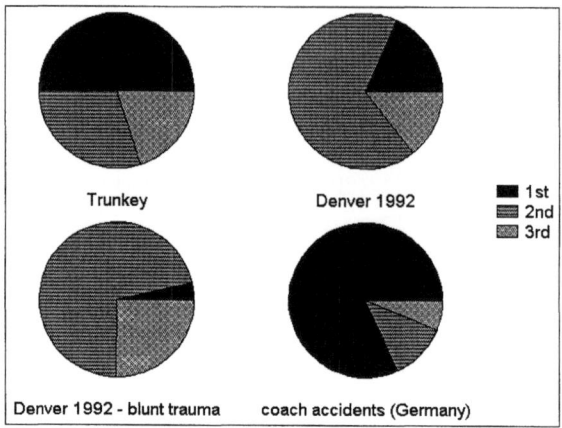

Figure 4.2: Trimodal distribution of death in different trauma systems

1st, 2nd, and 3rd refer to the three modes of trauma death. Trunkey: trimodal distribution of death as described by Trunkey, 1983[252], representing a 'scoop & run' system in transition between combination hearses/ambulances and paramedic care. Denver, 1992: All trauma deaths of the City and County of Denver, Colorado, 1992 (advanced life support by paramedics), blunt trauma — data of victims of blunt trauma only[221]. Coach accidents (Germany): Decade from 1992 to 2001. 'Treat & run' physician-based trauma system. From table 4.3, page 39

First basic and advanced life support ambulance systems were introduced, but especially in rural areas the 'funeral director' with a combination vehicle (hearse and ambulance) still provided emergency ambulance cover[183]. The paramedic emergency medical system in Denver did worse. Its performance in blunt trauma is even poorer. The limits of paramedic advanced life support in trauma patients have been recognized frequently (Table 4.4, page 43). The German coach accident victims show a different picture. The low second and third modes of trauma deaths show the same effectiveness of prehospital care as the success in the resuscitation after out of hospital cardiac arrest. The quality

> *"Paramedic rapid sequence intubation protocols to facilitate intubation of head-injured patients were associated with an increase in mortality and decrease in good outcomes" (USA)*[67]
>
> *"It was surprising that the outcome was almost always fatal" (intubation, UK)*[160]
>
> *"Prehospital intubation is associated with a significant increase in morbidity and mortality in trauma patients with traumatic brain injury" (USA)*[38]
>
> *"Prehospital endotracheal intubation appears to offer no demonstrable survival or functional advantage" (USA)*[61]
>
> *"The aggregated data in the literature have failed to demonstrate a benefit for on-site ALS provided to trauma patients and support the scoop and run approach" (meta-analysis, Canada)*[155]
>
> *"Patients with severe trauma transported by private means in this setting have better survival than those transported via the EMS system" (USA)*[68]

Table 4.4: Limitations of paramedic advanced life support

of the physician provided immediate care of the German trauma system had already been recognized by Trunkey[252]. A comparison between a German physician-staffed (Hanover) and an American nurse/ paramedic manned (Knoxville, Tennessee) helicopter emergency system found a statistically significant higher number of early deaths in the American system[223]. The widely disparate results can be seen as representative for the three systems of prehospital trauma care (haphazard, paramedic, emergency physician). They form a useful basis for auditing the management of mass casualty incidents.

4.3.2 Trimodal Distribution of Death in Major Incidents

The trimodal distribution of trauma death as an audit tool is applied to different types of major incidents: To burns, aircrashes,

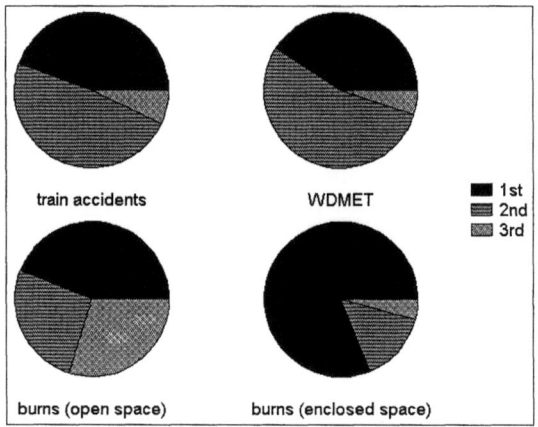

Figure 4.3: Trimodal distribution of death in different disaster scenarios
1st, 2nd, and 3rd refer to the modes of the trimodal distribution.
Data from tables 4.5, 4.6, and 4.7, pages 46, 47, and 48. For
comparison outcomes of military medicine: WDMET — Wound
Data and Munitions Effectiveness Team (combat fatalities in the
Vietnam war 1967 – 1969)[246]. Note the difference between the
burns sustained in open and enclosed spaces

and explosions to build a data base to compare to the Ramstein
airshow incident, and to train crashes for a comparison to the
high speed train crash at Eschede. Data from the Vietnam war
(WDMET — Wound Data and Munitions Effectiveness Team
(combat fatalities 1967 – 1969)[246]) put the results into perspective.
Incidents involving numerous burns casualties are divided into
those which occured in open and enclosed spaces. In the latter,
the severely injured are often unable to escape to the outside and
perish in the flames[173]. Noto's concept of the 'polyaggression
syndrome' ('brûlé, blasté, blessé' — combination of burns, blast,
and other major injuries) [192] justifies combining aircrashes, bombs,
other explosions, major fires, and similar incidents as their path-
omechanical consequences are comparable.

Methods

Case reports and documentations of major incidents involving train accidents, open, and enclosed fire, explosion, or aircrash incidents were identified using medline, embase, www search engines (metager.de, google), and a hand search of relevant journals and books. Inclusion criteria were:
Either train accidents or fire/explosion/aircrash potentially leading to polyaggression syndrome
Multiple casualties: $\geq$ 10 casualties
Severity: Impact severe enough to cause mortality
Survivability: At least one casualty survives the impact
Clear account of incident published, the trimodal distribution of death can be identified
Location and time: any

Results

Reports of 17 train accidents fulfilled the inclusion criteria (table 4.5, page 46). For mass casualty incidents involving patients with polyaggression syndrome, 14 incidents in open and 34 in enclosed spaces were identified (tables 4.6, 4.7, pages 47, 48).

Discussion

Figure 4.3, page 44, shows distributions of trauma death similar to the original description by Trunkey, rather than to the distributions of more advanced emergency medical systems. Given that the incidents occured in 21 countries in four continents, it is not surprising, that the results come closest to those of the 'haphazard' trauma system of Trunkey. The distribution of victims after burns/explosions in enclosed spaces shows a limit of the model: Those who are able to get out alive stay alive. Those who are severely injured are unable to escape, leading to an extremely high first mode. This reproduces the result of Mackie and Koning[173] that

year	country	dead	1st	2nd	3rd	injured	source
2003	Germany	6	6	0	0	25	21
2002	Austria	6	6	0	0	16	76
2002	UK	7	4	2	1	75	14, 17, 16, 20
2002	Portugal	5	4	1	0	7	18
2002	South Africa	22	6	12	4	117	15, 8, 13
2002	USA	2	1	1	0	265	19
2000	Germany	9	8	0	1	143	230
2000	Czech Republic	1	0	1	0	14	9, 10
1999	Germany	2	2	0	0	33	5
1999	Germany	5	3	2	0	44	71
1997	Germany	6	6	0	0	13	109
1995	Germany	1	0	1	0	57	265
1992	Germany	11	7	4	0	62	182
1990	Germany	17	16	0	1	86	91
1988	UK	35	33	1	1	119	247
1975	UK	45	21	20	2	70	3
1952	UK	112	6	96	10	287	250

Table 4.5: Major train accidents

1st, 2nd, and 3rd refer to the modes of the trimodal distribution of trauma deaths

indoors fire disasters lead to a large number of immediate deaths while outdoors fires result in a large number of severely injured. Nearly half of the incidents in the analysis come from European countries with strong physician involvement in prehospital care, a rather small area of the world. This reflects a particular publication bias: Many reports of fire disasters from outside these countries could not be assessed regarding the trimodal distribution of death. Their authors did not describe the mortality in sufficient detail, often providing the total number of deaths or the number of in hospital fatalities only. They seem to limit themselves to their particular area only, be it the ambulance service, the emergency department, or specialist/intensive care. What happens outside these narrow boundaries seems to be 'none of their business'. The European prehospital emergency doctors see and describe patient care from the scene of the accident to the intensive care unit as

year	country	type of incident	dead	1st	2nd	3rd	injured	source
2003	USA	explosion	6	3	0	3	≈ 20	243
2000	Netherlands	explosion	18	18	0	0	947	124, 229
1996	USA	bomb	2	0	2	0	110	85
1995	USA	aircrash	10	1	2	7	19	213
1994	USA	aircrash	15	9	2	4	115	211
1992	Greece	BLEVE	14	1	0	13	21	128
1988	Germany	aircrash	6	6	0	0	50	87
1988	Israel	bomb	6	3	1	2	52	142
1987	Germany	BLEVE	6	2	1	3	47	235
1984	Mexico	BLEVE	690	300	250	140	≈ 2000	28
1980	Germany	bomb	13	12	0	1	200	167
1979	Romania	explosion	48	2	2	44	47	1
1978	Spain	BLEVE	208	102	15	91	35	25
1974	UK	explosion	11	4	0	7	8	130

Table 4.6: Mass burn incidents and explosions in open spaces
BLEVE = boiling liquid expanding vapour explosion. 1st, 2nd, and
3rd refer to the modes of the trimodal distribution of trauma deaths

a continuum. The prehospital doctors, often anaesthetists, will
hand over the patients to their anaesthetic/ITU colleagues in the
resuscitation room, and are likely to meet the patients again when
they are rostered for duties in ITU, in the operating theatres, or
an acute pain round. This continuity of care is reflected in the
reports.
The trimodal distribution of trauma deaths is a valid tool to audit
outcomes after major incidents. Different types of disaster lead
to similar distributions (war, train accidents, burns/explosions
in open spaces). It is not suitable for analysing burns/explosion
incidents in enclosed spaces.

year	country	type of incident	dead	1st	2nd	3rd	injured	source
2001	Switzerland	aircrash	24	24	0	0	9	136
2000	Germany	explosion	12	11	0	1	25	231
2000	Germany	house fire	1	0	1	0	26	37
1999	Austria	explosion	9	9	0	0	2	248
1998	Germany	house fire	1	1	0	0	26	120
1996	Germany	airport fire	17	16	0	1	62	172
1996	Germany	arson	10	9	1	0	39	226
1996	Italy	BLEVE	5	5	0	0	34	177
1995	Germany	house fire	2	2	0	0	12	141
1995	France	bomb	3	2	1	0	63	217
1995	USA	bomb	168	164	4	0	≈ 700	122
1994	Germany	bomb	6	2	4	0	8	63
1994	Japan	aircrash	264	255	6	3	7	140
1994	Denmark	explosion	6	4	0	2	15	79
1993	USA	bomb	6	5	0	1	1042	158
1992	France	aircrash	87	81	6	0	9	140
1989	Canada	aircrash	24	22	0	2	45	140
1989	USA	aircrash	112	111	0	1	171	139
1989	UK	aircrash	47	39	4	4	79	219
1988	France	aircrash	3	3	0	0	36	140
1987	Spain	bomb	27	21	0	6	39	137, 98
1986	Germany	bomb	2	1	1	0	2000	267
1985	UK	stadium fire	60	55	0	5	78	28
1985	UK	aircraft fire	53	52	0	1	84	195
1983	Lebanon	bomb	241	234	1	6	105	95
1983	USA	aircraft fire	23	23	0	0	23	139
1981	India	circus fire	180	92	71	17	≈ 500	28
1977	Spain	aircrash	583	574	0	9	61	138
1976	USA	aircrash	37	37	0	0	35	138
1975	UK	bomb	1	0	0	1	36	254
1974	USA	aircrash	93	87	0	6	4	138
1974	UK	bomb	2	0	1	1	80	263
1972	UK	aircrash	118	117	1	0	0	138
1942	USA	fire	491	150	295	46	125	220

Table 4.7: Mass burn incidents, aircrashes, and explosions in enclosed spaces
BLEVE = boiling liquid expanding vapour explosion. 1st, 2nd, and
3rd refer to the modes of the trimodal distribution of trauma deaths

Chapter 5

The Ramstein Air Show Disaster 1988

The air show incident was unique: No other disaster has given rise to such controversy or shown such a clash of cultures of emergency management. It was a major political problem right from the outset.

The frank and open, often very controversial discussions typical of the German society and its emergency services contrasted with military secrecy.

'Freedom of speech', 'open government', and active parliamentary oppositions at state and federal level dragged every unpleasant detail into the public discussion. Numerous allegations of poor preparation and mismanagement were made. Debates in the federal[69] and in the state[153] parliaments and the findings of an enquiry commission of the federal parliament[33] are a good source for such allegations and problems which are rarely discussed in detail in more sober medical publications[175, 80, 149, 268, 232].

While not all allegations can be refuted or verified 15 years later, they reflect the chaos of the incident and contributed to the thought processes in the German emergency medical community.

Only this very open debate gave the German emergency services the opportunity to reassess their capabilities and introduce change.

5.1 The Incident

On the 28th August 1988 the US Airbase at Ramstein, state of Rhineland-Palatia, Germany, hosted an international airshow. More than 300 000 spectators gathered to watch the displays of the air forces of seven nations.

During a performance ('pierced heart maneuvre') by the Frecce Tricolori (Italian Air Force acrobatics team) three of their ten jet aircraft collided. Two planes crashed onto the airfield destroying a US Air Force medevac helicopter. The third plane fell into the crowd of spectators and exploded on hitting the ground. Burning fast-food vans with exploding propane gas bottles added to the conflagration.

The emergency services were faced with numerous dead and more than 500 injured.

5.2 Preparation

The 316th Air Division of the US Air Force Europe (USAFE) hosted the event. Emergency preparations for the airshow were kept under US Air Force control without any major involvement of German authorities who probably were considered suspect after an unanimous resolution by the Kaiserslautern County Council in 1984 asking for an immediate stop to airshows at Ramstein.

Medical care, fuel supplies, transport, etc were the responsibility of the 'logistics' operational element. Separate preparations for major incidents and for crowd care allowed the US Air Force to avoid having to comply with host nation standards of disaster control.

The medical management of major incidents stayed under American control without involvement of German agencies at state or federal level.

For the medical care of the spectators the organiser hired the Red Cross association of Kaiserslautern as a private agency two months before the event. In the previous years this arrangement had been satisfactory for caring for the many patients with heat exhaustion, medical problems, and minor cuts and bruises. The local Red Cross association provided seven doctors, 90 (mainly volunteer) helpers (ranging from first aiders to nurses and paramedics), one mobile intensive care unit, a speed intervention car, two basic life support ambulances, and a mobile first aid station.

The USAFE provided 14 doctors, 82 other medical corps staff, 9 ambulances (presumably basic life support), and three ambulance helicopters (not staffed by doctors). Two of the ambulances and one helicopter (which later got destroyed by falling debris) formed a disaster response team.

Outside the airfield, the Red Cross had three doctors, 25 helpers, and nine ambulances on standby.

The US Army Regional Medical Center at Landstuhl ($\approx$ 5km south of Ramstein, 260 beds, $\approx$ level 2 trauma centre) with an additional ambulance helicopter was put on alert for a possible major incident.

The plan was for the German Red Cross to treat German spectators, while the Americans would treat their own staff and provide cover for major incidents.

Four first aid stations were erected. Each had a German and an American section back to back, to enable handover of patients who by accident entered the wrong side.

The commander of the airfield base clinic was in overall command of all medical resources. Apparently this commander did not speak German, did not have much of an idea about the capabilities of the host nation emergency medical service, and did not liaise with the medical incident officers of the region.

A liaison officer kept the contact with the site command of the Red Cross.

This contrasts with 'security', an operational element in its own right, 800 US military police supported by 495 police officers of the state police of Rhineland-Palatia. The risk of disturbances by peace activists was obviously considered more serious than that of a major incident[69].

The county council of Kaiserslautern felt that additional precautions were necessary. It had deployed a part of its civil defence/major incident command ('gold command') to Miesenbach, the next village. An American liaison officer attended on request of the senior administrative officer of the county (head of 'gold command').

The council had warned the regional trauma centres, including the burns centre at the Ludwigshafen accident hospital. Emergency services, aid organisations, and civil defence agencies were asked to prepare for a possible major incident.

In previous years joint American and German disaster exercises had taken place. Their main focus seemed to have been firefighting and dealing with hazardous materials. The personnel of the German civilian emergency medical services could not remember attending any joint exercises of mass casualty management when questioned afterwards by the enquiry commissions of the federal and state parliaments.

5.3   Chaos on Scene and in the Hospitals

The aircrash caused a large conflagration involving numerous spectators. The air base fire service managed to control the fire within minutes.

Chaos ensued quickly. Some spectators were stampeding away and some towards the scene. It soon became apparent that of the more than 500 victims many were children or adolescents. They had moved to the front of the crowd to see the air performances instead of just the backs of the grown-ups. Now they had been hit first.

Initially, no obvious incident command was evident. Spectators, the Red Cross, and American troops started to provide first aid. The Red Cross command noticed that the American liaison officer had disappeared. They were unable to make contact with the USAFE medical command – they could not find the command centre, it was no longer where it had been. Subsequently, no joint operations could take place because of a total lack of communications.

In the meantime, the Air Force had activated its incident plan. This apparently entailed relocating the command centre and 'forgetting' about the German Red Cross — they were not part of the disaster response anyway. All casualties were to be transported to the emergency department at the US hospital in Landstuhl, by any means of transport, without treatment at the scene.

Both the German police and the Red Cross called the county incident command and ambulance control. It is unclear when the USAFE incident commander asked for host nation support, it appears this did not happen straight away.

When the first civilian immediate care doctors, helicopters, advanced, and basic life support ambulances arrived, they did not find a medical incident officer or any form of incident command to report to. Attempts at creating a command structure and a triage area failed, when civilians and soldiers carrying casualties on makeshift stretchers overran the arriving vehicles and forced them to transport their patients. The anaesthetist of the Christoph 5 air ambulance (Ludwigshafen trauma centre) reported: "We were able to provide immediate care, e.g. infusions, analgesia, for 10 – 15 patients, until some military transport helicopters landed near by. This influenced events: Now started a hectic, headless, utterly planless loading of casualties into these machines. We were unable to exert any influence on this and it was done in such a hectical way that e.g. venous cannulae were ripped out"[268]. To the German responders the US military seemed to have degenerated into a mob. Patients were transported on the back of pickup trucks, in ambulances, buses, lorries, and helicopters. A survivor graphically describes how he was put on the back of a US Air Force pickup truck together with four children and another adult[174].

Most casualties were transported to Landstuhl initially, both to LARMC and to the civilian St Johannis hospital, a rural general hospital. The latter, a small level 3 trauma centre, received ≈ 120 casualties. The patients loaded into German civilian ambulances and helicopters were distributed to a number of civilian trauma centres in the region.

Organized triage did not take place at the scene, only at the emergency department in Landstuhl. Some civilian immediate care doctors attempted to triage patients on the airfield, but were hindered by US soldiers. Inappropriate treatment of hopeless patients and undertreatment of salvageable casualties followed. One immediate care doctor even attempted to resuscitate a patient suffering a cardiac arrest during transport. The regional burns centres were flooded with burns patients with a poor prognosis. Patients with survivable burns were treated in general intensive care units even though they would have profited most from specialist care.

After 96 minutes the scene was cleared of casualties.

The access roads were blocked soon by visitors leaving the area, people with minor injuries seeking help elsewhere, people coming to the airfield to search for missing friends and relatives, and the curious.

Helicopters became extremely useful in these conditions. A total of 18 military and civilian helicopters doing several return flights each were involved in casualty evacuation.

It soon became obvious that the disaster had been shifted from the airfield to the two Landstuhl hospitals. In most patients treatment had not been started in the field and would not be initiated in the Landstuhl emergency rooms for several hours. Now patients were redistributed, reaching a total of 21 hospitals on the first day.

A federal army CH 53 ambulance helicopter brought eight doctors and burns supplies to Landstuhl. On the return flight, five patients with severe burns were taken to the burns centre at the federal army hospital in Koblenz.

US staff filled two buses with 43 and 22 casualties, and sent them to the university hospital in Homburg and to the regional burns centre in Ludwigshafen. The first bus got 'caught' by German police and escorted to its destination, the other lost its way and took over two hours to arrive. Both buses were full of apparently untriaged patients, many unstable.

At the receiving hospitals, doctors were surprised to find patients arriving without warning, without any documentation, some without any treatment, others with intravenous access and fluid giving sets incompatible to the ones in ordinary use. Other regional trauma centres did not receive casualties.

Many patients were redistributed subsequently to a total of 46 burns and trauma centres, including hospitals in Belgium, France, and the United States.

5.4 Lessons Learned

Here was a most sobering reality check for an emergency medical system considered one of the best of the world.

The usual 'pat on the back' for the emergency services was greated with derision: 'Unwilling to learn from the mistakes'. The problems and shortcomings had been too obvious.

The incident at Ramstein was one of those which could not be overlooked. Together with the aircrash at Remscheid and the boiling liquid expanding vapour explosion of a petrol tanker at Herborn it created sufficient pressure both on the medical community to change the approach to major incident management, and, at least as important, on the politicians to provide adaequate funding.

The German tendency to be outspoken to the brink of being impolite, the much beloved 'freedom of speech', frank, open discussion of the events, of mistakes, of responsibilities, and of the action to be taken allowed the identification of problems and solutions. The main lesson was that 'chaos kills'. Command and control were an important area for improvement.

A systematic approach to back up the emergency medical service was required.

The process of medical incident management had failed and needed review.

Psychological injuries, like post-traumatic stress disorder, became recognized widely.

5.4.1 Command and Control

Command and control, or the lack of it, was the main problem.

The lack of a unified command structure led to major chaos. Germans soon realized that their country had 'sovereignty deficits' with regards to the US allies/occupying forces who could disregard local arrangements and law. At Ramstein there was no medical incident officer, because the disaster plan of the state of Rhineland-Palatia was not binding on an area normally 'off limits to all Germans'.

The local county had established its 'gold command' incident command post in a nearby village. Unfortunately, no 'silver command' could be established on site, and the communication with the USAFE chain of command was lost early.

Cultural differences and language barriers further complicated the cooperation with foreign elements. Joint planning and preparation would probably have avoided most problems. A 'scoop & swoop' ideology in a 'stay & stabilise' system was doomed to fail. Prior planning for the establishment of an advanced medical post might have allowed an integration of both systems.

Weak leadership and a lack of communication before and during the incident both by the German civilian disaster control/emergency services and by the USAFE medical services caused poor coordination of available resources. With 800 US military police and 495 German state police officers it should have been possible to structure the scene, provide cordons, and clear access roads.

Command structures and incident officers need to be clearly identified and known to everybody involved in the incident response. Incident command must be established by the first emergency medical team on scene, handed over to trained incident officers as soon as possible, and reinforced by command support, with adaequate communications equipment.

5.4.2 Backup and Reserves

Own reserves: Prepared reserves both of the Red Cross and the USAFE were quickly deployed. Fire fighters of the airbase fire service and local volunteer fire departments provided useful first aid. Eight doctors, 15 nurses, and many first aiders could be recruited from the crowd of spectators. The widespread first aid training of the population (e.g. compulsory for applicants for driving licences) proved useful. The Kaiserslautern county ambulance service mobilised its immediate care doctors, advanced, and basic life support ambulances rapidly.

Mutual aid was activated without delay. Ambulance controls of other counties and the neighbour state of Saar did sent available helicopters, immediate care doctors, advanced, and basic life support ambulances. Initially, arriving units did not find a command structure to report to and were forced to participate in uncontrolled evacuation from the scene. At some point, ambulance control declared that further support was not needed, even though the LARMC intended to sent patients to distant hospitals by bus (not coordinated with ambulance control).

Helicopters: A total of 18 helicopters were used for patient transport, both fully equipped air ambulances and simple transport helicopters. While German air ambulances, both civilian and military, transported their patients to fairly distant trauma centres, the other helicopters were used for a Vietnam style 'scoop & swoop' operation, ferrying patients to the Landstuhl Army Regional Medical Center. The emergency room of this small hospital was also the main destination of ground ambulances and other vehicles used for patient transport and became overwhelmed soon. The large capacity CH 53 air ambulance of the federal army transported a team of eight immediate care doctors to the LARMC and on return flew five critically ill casualties to the burns centre at the Koblenz federal army hospital under full monitoring and intensive treatment.

Civil defence: 96 minutes after the crash the scene had been cleared of casualties. The civil defence medical platoons were presumably still in the process of alert by telephone snowballing at that point. Staff and equipment specially provided for major incident management could not give any useful contribution because the civil defence units were far too slow. Red Cross volunteers with similar or even less training had used their skills to good effect, because they had been on scene or standing by.

This lesson was learned: 55 rapid response teams were formed in the state of Rhineland-Palatia[92]. A skill mix ranging from civil defence aidmen to paramedics and immediate care doctors, equipment to normal peacetime standards, and fast alerts by radio pager enable these teams of volunteers and off-duty professionals to set up an advanced medical post in a realistic timeframe of 30 – 45 minutes after callout. Such a disciplined team will help structure the scene and allow other ambulance teams to integrate their efforts instead of stampeding to the next hospital.

5.4.3 Management of Major Incidents

The two basic principles of disaster management, triage and dispersal, seemed to have been applied only haphazardly. The mental models of incident management were incompatible, 'scoop & swoop' did not fit in with 'triage and dispersal'.

The 'scoop & swoop' tactics prevailed. The disaster was transferred into the receiving hospitals, especially the two hospitals at Land-stuhl. Transport before triage seemed the norm. Attempts at establishing triage areas by civilian immediate care doctors failed. Casualties with severe burns were undertriaged. The START algorithm fails these patients, labeling them 'green'/ T3, as they are often able to walk initially. It is unclear whether all patients had been triaged by doctors at the LARMC or whether patients had been triaged by protocol-based healthcare professionals only, before they were transported by bus to regional trauma and burns centres. For the walking wounded T3 patients bus transport without prior stabilisation would have appeared appropriate, but these patients were not really the walking wounded, they had severe burns. Dynamic, repeated triage should have picked up these patients before they had deteriorated.

Hopeless patients were transported to burns centres first, blocking ITU beds for salvageable casualties. Triage on the scene could have avoided this[151]. Most patients did not have triage labels or any documentation of the treatment received.

The incident command was unable to account for the patients, e.g how many or who had been transported where. Simple triage card systems could have helped to control this chaos.

The single point of contact for burns centres, the Hamburg fire/ambulance control worked well. Instead of each individual receiving hospital trying to contact the regional burns centres, the Hamburg fire/ambulance control was able to allocate patients to centres all over Germany and abroad.

5.4.4 Post-Traumatic Stress Disorder

Psychological injuries both to the victims and the helpers became a huge problem. A team of doctors and psychologists started a group providing care[132]. Before this incident emergency planners had not often considered the need for aftercare. After Ramstein, psychosocial aftercare became a large and influential movement, involving churches, doctors, psychologists, social workers, and lay volunteers. Their methods are mainly based on Mitchell's concept of critical incident stress management. Evidence of effectiveness is still lacking, but the movement is by now very influential. Aftercare both of injured and uninjured victims and helpers is now an accepted standard of care.

5.5 Applying the Audit Tool

5.5.1 Structural Quality

The structural quality of the emergency medical service of any
given German area is usually high (table 5.1, page 61). Large
numbers of ground ambulances and immediate care doctors can
be mobilized through mutual aid. Helicopters travel at a speed
of 200–250 km/h, and are staffed by doctors and paramedics with
ample trauma experience.

In densely populated areas like most European countries, numerous
trauma centres are within this range. Dispersal of casualties is a
realistic option. In this incident, the civilian hospital at Landstuhl,
a small level 3 trauma centre, and the Landstuhl Army Regional
Medical Center received more than a hundred patients each, creating battlefield conditions. Other regional hospitals did not receive
any casualties. Distribution over the whole region would have
resulted in 10 or less patients per hospital. Individual medicine
and definitive care could have been provided earlier.

The weak point of Kaiserslautern county in 1988 was the provision
of an advanced medical post. The county relied on the poorly
functional and slow civil defence medical platoon. In the meantime,
this has been rectified and Kaiserslautern county got four rapid
response teams, three of which are able to set up an advanced
medical post, the fourth specialises in the welfare care of the
uninjured.

5.5.2 Process Quality

Looking at the processes, Ramstein looks like a joint German-
American effort to disregard any sound principles of incident management (table 5.2, page 62). What went surprisingly well was the
learning of lessons afterwards. Col. Paul, senior medical advisor to

standards and measures	
Regular emergency services: Availability of emergency doctors, helicopters ALS, and BLS ambulances within 15, 30, and 60 min (radius of 10/20/40 km (ground) or 50/100/200 km(air))	doctors: 1/4/17 helicopters: 3/5/11 ALS units: 2/9/57 BLS units: 3/18/54
rapid response teams within 20/40 km	not yet formed
state disaster units/civil defence within 20/40 km	medical platoon: 0/1
military/ other support within 60 min	SAR helicopter
standard: 1 doctor for 5 patients	Required: ≈ 115 doctors Available initially: Red Cross: 10 USAF: 14 spectators: 8 subsequently:≈ 10 –15 total: ≈ 50–55 one doctor for 10 patients
standard: 1 'helper' (from paramedic to civil defence aidman) for 1 patient	Required: ≈ 570 available initially: Red Cross: 115/USAF: 82 subsequently:≈ 100 total: ≈300 1 helper for 2 patients but 1300 policemen for ≈ 50 peaceniks
qualification of aid personnel	wide range
medical command structure: medical incident officer ambulance incident officer	established in county, not wanted by USAFE —
command support	—
advanced medical post: team and equipment	base clinic, 4 first aid posts civil defence medical platoon
trauma centers (level 1 – 3) within a distance of 30/60 minutes by ground/ by air	By ground 30/60 min: level 1 1/3 level 2 1/9 level 3 1/8 by air: level 1 7/11 level 2 38/>100
burns beds within 60 minutes	29

Table 5.1: Audit standards of structural quality

Data from (75, 81) and the parliamentary enquiries

standards and measures	
first team does not start treatment	they transported instead
provides short feedback to control	Red Cross volunteers did
gains an overview	did not happen
establishes command & control	command & control lost early
first command: "transport stop" — no spontaneous, uncontrolled transports to hospitals	not given many
reserves: time for control to mobilize backup were mutual aid, rapid response teams, disaster units, civil defence, the military, and independent providers called early? not enough or too many reserves mobilized?	 short, some backup on standby mutual aid yes German military yes initially not enough
triage use of established categories initial, e.g. START flexible, adapted to situation or protocol-based? dynamic, repeated over-/undertriage	 unclear, poorly documented most patients coming from LARMC did not have triage tags no, transport before triage — once at German hospitals yes undertriage of burns patients (probably because of START) patients with 90% burns sent to burns units blocking beds for salvageable casualties

Table 5.2: Audit standards of process quality

Continued overleaf

the federal armed forces, considered the emergency management to be 'phantastic' and 'excellent'. No lessons to be learned there. Fortunately he faced hoots and laughter by those willing to employ critical thinking. The latter attitude prevailed, and the German mass casualty incident system underwent major changes.

5.5.3 Outcome Quality

A total of 74 patients died as a consequence of the incident. 25 died immediately, a further 9 before evacuation from the airfield.

standards and measures	
stabilisation of 'immediate' patients before transport	no ('scoop & swoop' approach)
inappropriate procedures, e.g. CPR	CPR did happen
handover to medical/ ambulance incident officers	—
communication sufficient, breakdown of radio network?	language problems liaison officer lost no communication between US and German command radio system failed different radio frequencies, no direct communication between civilian and military agencies
advanced medical post established	not established
ambulance waiting area	not established
no self-deployment of ambulances/ teams ('disaster tourism')	did happen
dispersal to different hospitals	to 21 hospitals, mainly to LARMC
number of secondary (hospital to hospital) transfers	many (patients in 21 hospitals on 1st day, 46 hospitals later)

Table 5.3: Audit standards of process quality (continued)

During transport and in the first hours in hospital 12 casualties died. 28 late deaths occured subsequently over the next days and weeks (figure 5.1, page 64).

The trimodal distribution of death does not at all look like the German trauma deaths. It is similar, if not worse, to the average of all burns deaths. The outcome appears rather suboptimal.

Wresch[268] plotted the intravenous fluids given in the first hours to burns patients arriving at the Ludwigshafen burns centre against the fluid requirements for resuscitation of 30 and 70% surface area burns. The amounts actually given were far less than those required even for 30% body surface area burns. Mortality was high.

The editor of the official civil defence medical handbook[240], Leo Koslowski, professor of surgery, university of Tübingen, denounced the medical management of the Ramstein incident as 'appalling' and 'utterly chaotic' shortly afterwards[153]. The audit tool indic-

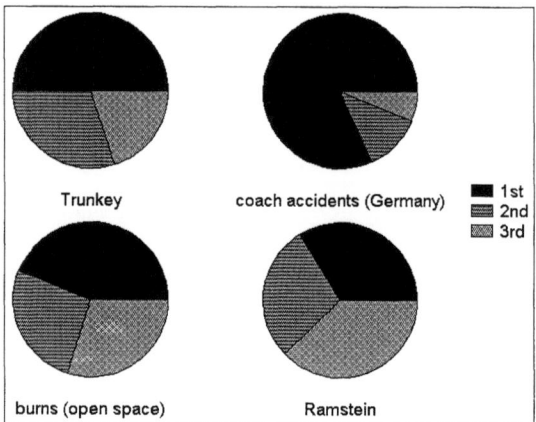

Figure 5.1: Trimodal distribution of death at the Ramstein incident

The distribution is worse than the average of comparable disasters supporting the widely held assumption that medical management had been substandard

ates he may have been right.

Chapter 6

Command and Control

6.1 The DV100 Incident Management System

6.1.1 Evolution of Incident Command

The air raid protection had a unified command system during the second world war: For civil defence the emergency services were integrated closely. All ambulance services were assimilated into the Red Cross. Fire services were integrated into the police forces ('fire protection police'). Voluntary fire brigades became auxiliary police departments. Fire protection police, Red Cross, and the technical aid service together formed the air raid protection police. Incident command lay with the most senior fire police officer supported by the integrated command and communication structures of fire protection and ordinary police. Officers usually had military staff college training and applied Clausewitz's ideas on strategy and operative tactics to dealing with major air raids[157, 107].

After the war, the command system was lost. The flood of 1962 was the first catastrophe to hit and overwhelm the resources of a total of four states. Clear command structures integrating the numerous agencies involved were missing. As such large incidents were rare, it obviously was easier to admire publicly the heroism of firefighters, civil defence workers, soldiers, and any number of others rather than asking nasty questions and drawing unwelcome conclusions.

The forest fires of 1975 in Lower Saxony again overwhelmed the state resources. Fire brigades and civil defence had to be supported by state police, the federal armed forces, border patrol, British allies/occupational forces, and French Canadair water bombers. The federal minister of the interior appointed a general of the (paramilitary) border patrol as the overall incident commander. The commander's lack of specialist knowledge, micromanagement of forward units, and political rather than technical priorities led to friction between overall and local command and 'suboptimal' cooperation between the different agencies involved. In the ensuing chaos five firefighters found their retreat cut off by rapidly spreading brushfire. They were not missed in time, wireless communications had broken down, helicopter search and evacuation was not requested, and all five perished in the flames. The lessons were learned.

6.1.2 The Command System

The agencies involved in major incident response have to speak the same language and have to be able to integrate themselves in a common command structure. Political, operational strategical, and tactical command need clearly separated areas of responsibility. All emergency response agencies including police and armed forces introduced the DV100 (Dienst-Vorschrift 100 = standing orders no. 100) incident management system[244, 212, 205]. This system recognizes three levels of command, allowing easy integration of a multitude of specialist agencies and departments (figure 6.1, page 70). At all three levels, functions can be filled by representatives of all emergency services (fire brigades, ambulance services, aid organisations, civil defence). The top level will always be headed by the senior administrative officer of the county/city and will assemble in prepared stations (e.g. county halls, with full communication equipment). The KatSL/disaster or 'gold' command is set up for large scale events affecting more than one site, e.g. floods, forest fires, accidents involving nuclear power stations, civilian unrest, or the ultimate disaster, war. 'Gold' command always works with full staff support, organized similarly to the staff of the 'silver' command (figure 6.2, 71). Only the head of the KatSL/disaster command may declare an area a 'disaster zone' with widespread legal implications.

Above the county 'gold' command the state or the federal government may occasionaly put higher levels of command for incidents involving many counties or more than one state (e.g. Oder floods). The middle level (TEL)[185] will be headed by a senior officer of a service with a major contribution to the management of the specific incident. Often this is a senior fire officer, in some circumstances it may be the medical incident officer or another specialist, e.g. mountain rescue at an avalanche. The TEL meets at a safe place near the incident, usually in command buses, tents, or fixed buildings quickly adapted for command, control, communication, and information. In some states, the TEL ('technical' command) is known as ÖEL (örtliche Einsatzleitung — local command).

The staff supporting the commander at top and middle level is organised in six staff functions S1–S6, and a panel of specialist advisors. The only differences between the staff of 'gold' and of 'silver' command are the support available to the staff officers and the composition of the advisory panel.

S1 (personnel) provides the manpower at an incident, alerts additional units, and builds reserves. Organizing critical incident stress management and/or pastoral care is also a S1 function.

S2 (situation) keeps 'situational awareness', supervises the drawing and updating of an event map, and takes care of documentation. This officer can be supported by reconnaissance teams.

S3 (action) deploys the available means. Through S3 the commander issues orders to the next lower level of command. Issuing orders directly to individual units is the task of the sector leaders ('bronze command'), not of higher command levels. Micromanagement stifling the initiative of frontline units is considered undesirable, in the tradition of Clausewitz tasks and information are given to lower levels who then are allowed to implement it in their own way. S4 (logistics) is responsible for supplies. Equipment, fuel, transport, medical supplies, etc. can be requested via S4, aid workers and the uninjured need food and shelter, ...

S5 (media) takes care of media relations, organizes press conferences, coordinates work with the media officers of other agencies, and acts as spokesperson for the command staff. This press/media liason officer is new, in the 1981 edition of the DV100 (official version at the Ramstein incident) this function did not yet exist.

S6 (communications) is another function added after Ramstein. Failures of radio and other communications occur frequently at major incidents. A specialist staff officer can either deal with or better help to avoid such problems.

The staff is supported by two panels of specialist advisors, internal and external. At 'gold' level, the internal advisors are representatives of the county's or city's own departments, e.g. public health, social services, housing, water, gas, and electricity supply (if provided by the county/city, if the utilities are delivered by private enterprises, they would be external advisors), public transport, fire department, environment office, road maintenance, etc. The external advisors are the liaison officers of the police, aid agencies, the military, privately run utilities, the railway, etc. At 'silver' level, the internal advisors are likely to be medical, ambulance, and fire incident officers, environment/hazardous materials specialists, a social services representative, etc, depending on the nature of the incident. External advisors would be the incident and liaison officers of police, border patrol, military, aid agencies, railways, utilities, airport or port authorities, factories, etc, activated on an as required basis.

Medical involvement in the command structures will vary according to need. At 'gold' level, a senior public health doctor is an internal specialist advisor. At 'silver' level, the medical incident officer may either be an internal advisor or the 'silver' commander, if the incident is mainly medical, e.g. mass poisoning, outbreaks of infectious diseases ...

At 'bronze' level, the medical incident officer (or another immediate care doctor if the medical incident officer is already working at 'silver' level) will be sector leader for e.g. an advanced medical post or immediate care in the accident area.

The levels of command are activated as needed. 'Bronze' or sector command is the everyday command at localized incidents, e.g. an immediate care doctor, a paramedic, and a fire/rescue officer coordinate the medical care and extrication of three entrapped casualties after a road traffic accident.

The middle level of command is called to major incidents. For example, at a crash of a jet airliner 'silver' command is established. It will be lead by the fire incident officer with full staff support, with the medical and the ambulance incident officer in the role of specialist advisors. Representatives of the police, the aid agencies, the airport authority, and the airline are part of the panel of external advisors. Several sectors will be formed, commanded by the most appropriate specialist officer, e.g. rescue of survivors (fire officer commanding rescue teams of the local fire brigade, a state disaster rescue unit, and the federal technical aid agency), firefighting (fire officer with local and airport fire units), advanced medical post (headed by an experienced immediate care doctor, with several medical teams, rapid response teams, and a state disaster control medical platoon), an ambulance waiting area (ambulance officer), a helicopter landing area (pilot of SAR helicopter), ...

'Gold' command will be put in place only at very major and widespread incidents, e.g. forest fires, floods, or an incident at e.g. a nuclear power station potentially involving large populated areas.

The Free State of Bavaria has recently introduced a command support team for the medical and ambulance incident officers, four experienced and trained men with a command van. The main

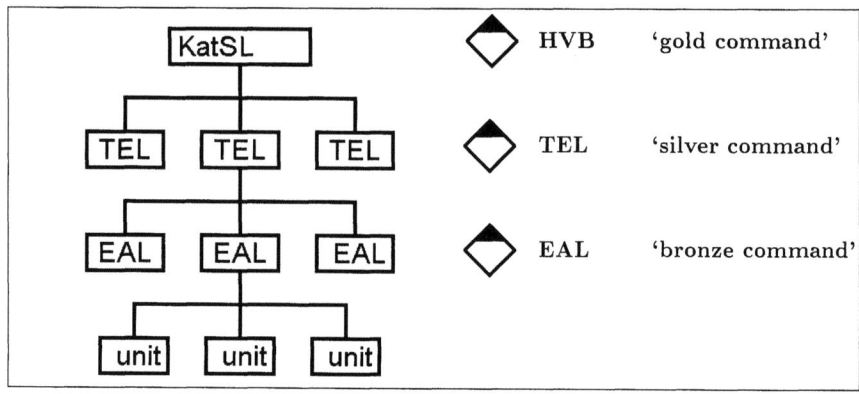

Figure 6.1: The DV100 incident command system

KatSL = Katastrophenschutzleitung ('gold command'), TEL = Technische Einsatzleitung/-leiter ('silver command', senior incident officer), EAL = Einsatzabschnittsleitung/-leiter ('bronze command', sector leader), HVB = Hauptverwaltungsbeamter (senior administrative officer of county). The HVB and the TEL usually lead with full staff support, the EAL is supported by a radio operator. The terms 'gold', 'silver', and 'bronze' command are not normally used in Germany. I have introduced them here to aid British readers

task is support with radio communications and documentation[144].
Other states will hopefully follow suit at some point.

6.2   LNA — Medical Incident Officer

The Leitender Notarzt (LNA/medical incident officer) is a key figure in mass casualty incident management.

The medical incident officer is alerted whenever coordination and leadership of the emergency medical services is required[166]:

– Incidents beyond the capacities of the regular emergency medical services

– Incidents endangering the health of a large number of persons

– On request by an immediate care doctor or an incident commander. Most counties have organised groups of medical incident officers (paid an on-call supplement), few still rely on unpaid volunteers[23].

70

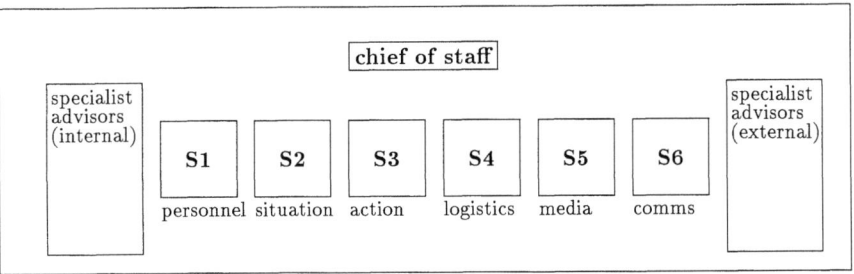

Figure 6.2: Structure of KatSL — disaster/'gold' command and TEL — technical/'silver' command

This trained team advises the senior administrative officer (HVB, 'gold commander') and the senior incident officer (TEL, 'silver commander'). The functions S1–6 are explained in the main text. A liaison officer of the British forces would be one of the 'external advisors' (right side of picture). Top/'gold' and middle/'silver' command differ in the specialist advisors and in the support available to the staff officers S1–6.

Joint recommendations of the German Interdisciplinary Association for Intensive Care (DIVI — deutsche interdisziplinäre Vereinigung für Intensivmedizin) and the federal chamber of physicians[44] regulate the selection (table 6.2, page 73) and training[90] (table 6.3, page 74) of medical incident officers[26, 152]. Refresher courses and updates help to maintain skills and knowledge[73, 74]. Most medical incident officers are anaesthetists[78], reflecting the base specialty of most immediate care doctors. The senior anaesthetist is considered the ideal candidate for medical incident officer training: Anaesthetists have experience in management and the setting of priorities in operating theatres and intensive care units, they are used to work in a team with a wide variety of different specialists, know the capacities of the regional intensive care units (a common bottleneck in major incidents) and emergency medical services and have a high credibility both in the prehospital and the hospital environment. Duty psychiatrists or orthopaedic surgeons, even if trained in a short course, do not have any role in medical

- evaluates the situation

  – tactical (type of incident, nature of injuries, number of casualties, intensity and size of damage, dangers of scene, additional hazards, likely developments)

  – own situation (staff, equipment, transport capacity, dangers and hazards, hospital capacities)

- decides upon the 'Schwerpunkt'/main focus of effort, and the nature of the emergency medical care (triage, medical care, transport)

- emergency medical care

  – determines priorities for treatment and transport

  – determines level of medical care

  – delegation of medical tasks

  – determines type of and need for patient transport

  – determines need for medical equipment

  – medical documentation

Table 6.1: Tasks and responsibilities of the medical incident officer

A lot to do for a single person. Most tasks will be delegated

command.

The emergency medical services command is formed jointly by the medical incident officer and the ambulance incident officer[203]. The former is mainly responsible for medical tactical decisions (table 6.1, page 72)[249]), the latter for organisational tactics. The medical incident officer has the right to give orders in all matters related to patient care.

The medical incident officer course has been adapted for international delegates. As most international candidates have little experience in prehospital immediate care, 'in field treatment' training has been added. This 'International Chief Emergency Physician Training Course on Mass Casualty Incidents' (ICEP) is run once yearly by the International Trauma Anaesthesia and Critical Care Society (ITACCS). Course dates are available on the ITACCS

- Certificate of completion of specialist training in an acute specialty with close involvement in critical care

- Certificate of competency in prehospital immediate care or equivalent

- Minimum of three years experience in prehospital immediate care

- Continuing participation in prehospital immediate care

- Minimum of six months full time training in intensive care

- medical incident officer training course (40h)

- Regular attendance at refresher courses and meetings

Table 6.2: Requirements for LNA/medical incident officers

web site (http://www.itaccs.com).

6.3 Organisatorischer Leiter/OrgL (Ambulance Incident Officer)

The OrgL/ambulance incident officer works closely with the medical incident officer. The main tasks of the ambulance incident officer are organization and logistics, the 'order of the space'/structuring the scene, requesting additional resources through ambulance control, and coordination between medical incident officer and ambulance control of the transport and distribution of patients[65]. The training is usually regulated at state level (one week course)[180].

The ambulance incident officer is usually either a senior fire officer where the emergency medical service is run by the fire brigade, or an experienced paramedic/ EMT-intermediate (ambulance station officer). Minimum qualifications are paramedic or EMT-intermediate training, five years experience, civil defence leadership training (at least section leader), and the training course.

- medical training

  - triage
  - medical care at a mass casualty incident

- legal basis and administrative structures

  - legal basis for the work of the medical incident officer
  - structure of disaster control
  - organizational structure of police, fire service, emergency medical service, and aid organisations

- tactical training

  - fundamentals of leadership and emergency medical care
  - coordination with other services
  - documentation

- technical training

  - equipment and vehicles for rescue and technical aid
  - communication and radio equipment

- exercises

  - several radio communications exercises
  - table top exercise: mass casualty incident
  - table top exercise: joint command in the DV100 incident management system
  - field exercise of a large-scale incident with local emergency services

Table 6.3: LNA/medical incident officer training course

For Euro 550 ($\approx$ £340) this 40 hour course looks good value. The syllabus hides the informal curriculum, handing down practical experiences of real-world incidents. Note the emphasis on radio communication skills, as breakdowns or overloads of radio communications are common problems at major incidents. No trauma training is given, the course delegates will have had ample experience in immediate care anyway. The final field exercise is used for assessment, e.g. a candidate who starts treating casualties instead of coordinating will fail. Such courses take place several times each year, course centres are accredited by the chambers of physicians

Chapter 7

Mobilising Support and Reserves

Major incidents are characterized by a demand for medical care far exceeding the available resources. The ability to mobilize reserves rapidly is a key factor in the successful management of mass casualty incidents. The medical incident command can mobilize:

local reserves

mutual aid

rapid response teams

state disaster units/civil defence

aeromedical services

military support

All these assets can be mobilized in a timely fashion. They will work within the framework of the DV100 incident command system. By training and equipment they can integrate themselves into the normal emergency medical system with its standard operating procedures.

Voluntary aid associations may provide rapid response teams or disaster units. Volunteers outside these trained units, e.g. those providing care at mass gatherings, are not normally considered worthwile reserves. Training may be insufficient, equipment variable, and response times several hours.

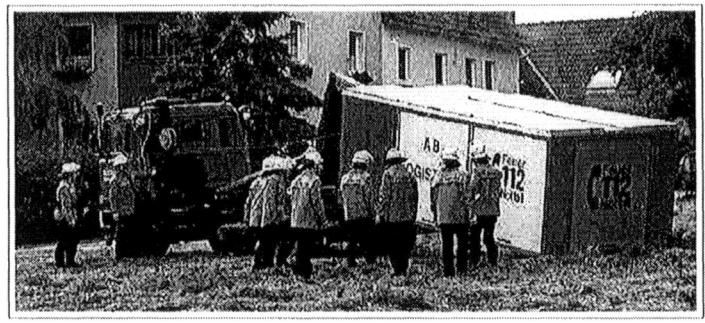

Figure 7.1: Container pod with tents and equipment for an advanced medical post

7.1 Local Reserves

The first back up available are local assets[171]. Basic life support ambulances are diverted from routine patient transports. Staffed by an EMT-intermediate and an EMT-basic, they provide an immediately available pool of trained personnel, equipment, and transport capacity. Professional fire brigades move firefighters/paramedics from fire fighting units to advanced life support ambulances. In cities where the fire department provides the ambulance service, firemen/paramedics on duty for e.g. water tenders routinely staff reserve advanced life support ambulances to cover peaks in demand for emergency medical services[181]. Large brigades are equipped with bus ambulances and prime movers carrying container pods of medical equipment (figure 7.1, page 76)[224, 179]. Together with the staff of a fire/rescue platoon — all trained to paramedic or at least EMT-intermediate level — an advanced medical post/casualty treatment station can be formed [242]. Aid organizations and other independent providers not involved in the official emergency medical service may provide professionally staffed advanced or basic life support ambulances which are available immediately. Depending on political persuasion, some places encourage the use of these assets, while areas with more left wing governments tend to ignore the resources of the 'private profiteers'. During normal working hours hospitals can provide additional immediate care doctors at short notice, e.g. by stopping routine operating lists and clinics.

7.2 Mutual Aid

Mutual aid from neighbouring counties and cities can be mobilized rapidly. Preexisting plans help the fire/ambulance controls in requesting an appropriate number of immediate care doctors, advanced, and basic life support ambulances. Depending on local resources, helicopters, rapid response teams, and state disaster control/civil defence units can also be called. Clear meeting points, ideally preplanned, and ambulance waiting areas help to integrate mutual aid into the larger plan. This is especially important for immediate care doctors and ALS ambulances coming directly from their individual stations. Mutual aid should not be deployed by its own fire/ambulance control without a request by the control of the incident area. In the border areas the mutual aid plans include cross-border help. Mutual aid will often be invoked without a major incident, to provide area cover during times of saturation of an emergency medical system.

7.3 Rapid Response Teams

Rapid response team = 'Schnelleinsatzgruppe' (SEG) or 'Sondereinsatzgruppe' (literally: special response team). In the last 15 years rapid response teams became an important part of major incident preparations. Their idea is based on an observation: If the regular, professional emergency medical service needed support, civil defence units could be called. Alerted by telephone snowballing, a large unit (medical platoon, figure 3.4, page 26) would turn up several hours later. Their training and equipment was substandard compared to the regular emergency medical services.

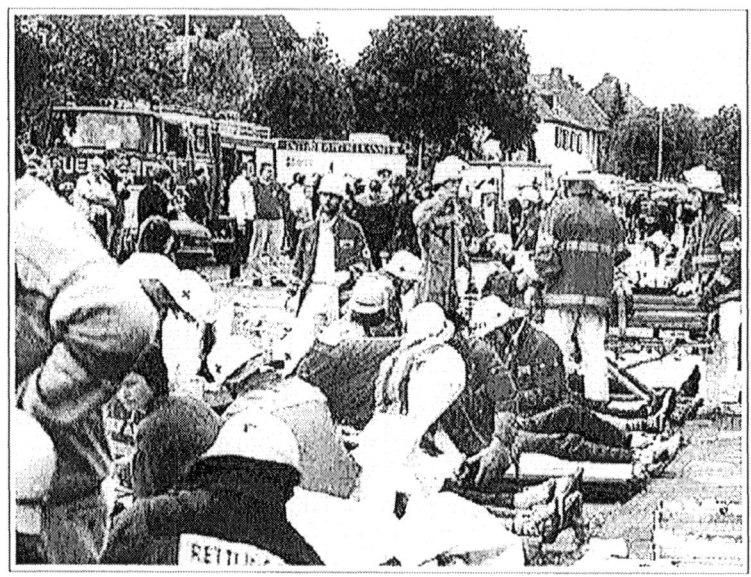
Figure 7.2: Rapid response team

If, on the other hand, a professional fire brigade needed support, volunteer fire brigades would be alerted by radio pager (or by siren signals in rural areas). Fifteen minutes later fire trucks would arrive, training and equipment designed to interface easily with any other fire brigade, paid professional or volunteer.

Soon the first units were formed along the lines of the volunteer fire brigades[224]: Radio pagers activated by ambulance control, advanced training geared towards cooperation with the regular emergency services, and modern equipment give a high tactical value. The staffing can be anything from off-duty doctors and paramedics to civil defence aidmen, often a mix of different skills. Team strength can vary between five and sixty members, most teams can reliably provide 10 – 20 trained 'helpers' at any time. Most teams tend to train their volunteer members to EMT-basic or intermediate level, with additional training in the management of major incidents[72]. Off-duty paramedics often act as their officers.

The size of these units can vary from small teams, equipped with a Volkswagen van, to large units with special custom-built vehicles, command cars, advanced, and basic life support ambulances[161]. Many teams upgrade civil defence vehicles to peacetime standards or adapt old fire engines.

The units are often affiliated to an aid association, some teams come from civil defence or state disaster units, others belong to an official or private ambulance service. Their main tasks are:

- staffing of reserve ALS and BLS ambulances

- setting up and running an advanced medical post

- support for triage and documentation

- on-site emergency medical care

- stretcher bearer teams

- organising an ambulance waiting area

- transport of emergency patients

- transport of supplies

- care of uninjured persons

- feeding and sheltering aid personnel and victims

- helping with the evacuation of hospitals, nursing homes, or other areas

- ...

Soon many teams realized that they were not able to provide all services to a high standard. Most teams now specialise in one area[198]:

- advanced medical post (SEG-Behandlungsplatz/Sanität)[106]

- emergency medical care in the disaster area (SEG-Rettung)

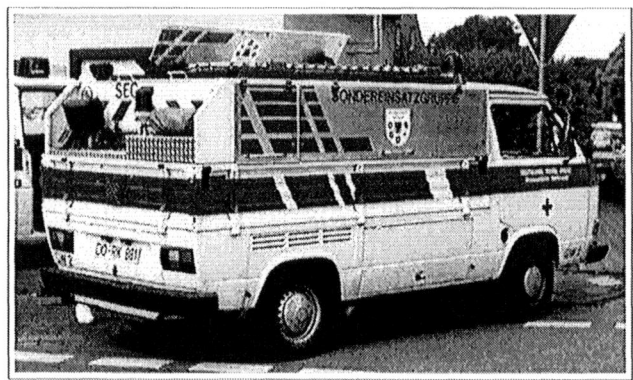

Figure 7.3: Equipment van of the rapid response team of the Red Cross in Dortmund

A command car, two equipment, and a staff van, 4x4 Volkswagen Synchro vans, transport team and equipment for an advanced medical post[224]

- patient transport (SEG-Transport)

- welfare/care of the uninjured (SEG-Betreuung)

- command support (SEG-Führungsunterstützung)

Rapid response teams are usually available 10 – 30 minutes after the alert.

Some teams have developed special expertise in dealing with hazardous materials/ decontamination of casualties[96].

Initially, there were concerns that civil defence aidmen were filling positions both in their own civil defence unit and in a rapid response team. This never seemed to be much of a practical problem and by simply redesigning the rapid response team as an 'advance party' the bureaucratic problem was solved[199].

7.4 State Disaster Units/Civil Defence

The main problems with civil defence and state disaster units were insufficient training and equipment, response times of several hours, and poor motivation of the national servicemen and volunteers.

This has improved markedly (see chapter 3). Now most units see themselves in the role of a rapid response team. Radio pagers supplanted telephone snowballing, the equipment is continuously modernised, and training made more relevant to the problems of today[104]. Most states sponsor training of former civil defence aidmen to EMT-basic or intermediate level.

With the improvements came more callouts, leading to more experience and higher morale. Providing help at a coach accident is more meaningful and gains more recognition than training for the nuclear holocaust of an unlikely 3rd World War.

Except for Brandenburg which designed its units completely from scratch (figure 3.6, page 32), most states either based their units on the old civil defence medical platoon or on the Red Cross model (figure 3.8, page 34). The latter is the combination of a medical and a welfare section, supported by a command squad and a technical squad. The medical section can either set up a small advanced medical post or add its capabilities to an existing advanced medical post. If required, it can be supported by the welfare section whose helpers are trained civil defence aidmen. The welfare section can take care of the uninjured and may be supported by the men of the medical section. The technical squad gives the unit a degree of autonomy (provision of electricity, light, repairs ...). Useful tasks for such a unit can be to take care of the walking wounded, assist at an advanced medical post, and help with patient transport either from the scene of an incident to an advanced medical post or from the latter to hospitals. Disaster control units take about 30 minutes to be ready for deployment.

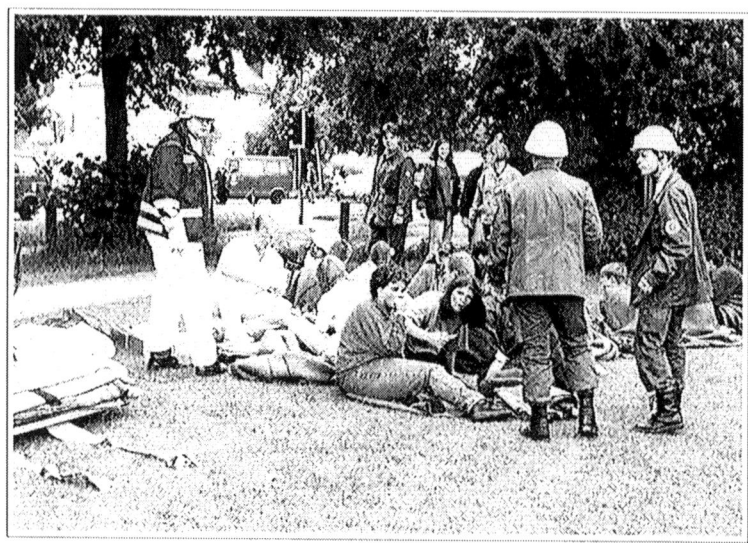

Figure 7.4: Aidmen of a disaster control unit
support a paramedic (left) in the care of casualties with minor injuries

7.5 Aeromedical Service

Helicopters play a major part in modern incident response[54, 266].
They have three main functions:

- air reconaissance of the scene

- rapid transport of highly experienced immediate care doctor/
  paramedic teams and equipment. The aeromedical service
  provides a fast and reliable reserve for immediate care doctors.

- aeromedical evacuation of critical casualties to distant trauma
  centres (dispersal), allowing each trauma centre to treat one
  or two polytrauma patients to normal standards of individual
  medicine.

Three overlapping nets of helicopter emergency medical services cover the whole of Germany:

- The network of Christoph helicopters (figure 2.7, page 16): The regular helicopter emergency medical service, described in chapter 2. 56 stations cover the whole of the nation in circles of 50 km diameter. Given a flight speed of 200 – 250 km/h, a large number of helicopters can be called together within 30 to 60 minutes.
  Most Christoph helicopters are available during daylight hours only. They start within two minutes of the alert.
  In border areas neighbourhood help works extremely well, and REGA helicopters (Switzerland), the Austrian Christopher and Martin machines, Christoph Lux (Luxembourg), the French SAMU helicopters, or the three HEMS stations in the Netherlands may be called via their respective controls.

- The second net is formed by the intensive care transfer helicopters. They are staffed by anaesthetists/intensivists and ITU nurses or specially trained paramedics[258]. The experienced team and the advanced equipment (e.g. ITU ventilator) come in handy to transfer ventilated patients to distant centres, e.g. intubated burns patients. The number of stations is less than for the primary helicopter emergency medical service, but in most state at least one or two ITU transfer helicopters are stationed.
  Many ITU helicopters have night-flight capability.

- The third net is provided by the military 'Search and Rescue' (SAR) helicopters[39]. Some stations are fully integrated into the Christoph helicopter emergency medical service, with helicopters equipped to civilian standards, staffed by immediate care doctors and paramedics. Helicopters without doctor, with a medical NCO (EMT-intermediate) cover thirteen other stations. If required, these helicopters can be 'medicalised' by taking up a doctor and equipment either at civilian or military hospitals or at the scene. The SAR helicopters are available 24 hours every day.

Large numbers of transport helicopters and fixed wing aircraft not normally involved in aeromedical services can be mobilized at some notice.

The federal armed forces provide a special support helicopter for major incidents at three stations. The CH 53G is staffed by three teams of immediate care doctors and paramedics. Equipped to a similar standard as the resuscitation room of a large hospital, the machine can transport up to five ventilated patients or 12 stretcher cases[29]. These helicopters are available within one hour of an alert.

Further transport helicopters can be provided by the paramilitary federal border patrol and by state police forces.

7.6 Military Support

The SAR helicopters and the large capacity CH 53G air ambulances are the most important military assets to support major incident management.

Other equipment, e.g. medical teams, ground ambulances, off-road ambulances, burn kits for 35 patients each, large numbers of aidmen and stretcher bearers, etc ... can be made available on request[147, 146].

Offers to help by NATO allies/occupational forces can be coordinated best by the federal armed forces. Liaison officers and interpreters can be provided rapidly, officers who know both the allies and the German civilian emergency system. If required, they can 'babysit' medical detachments of NATO allies turning up at the scene of a major incident, help with communication and translation, ensure that treatment provided is not substandard, stop uncoordinated transportation of casualties by non-German units, and generally avoid chaos to prevent another Ramstein.

Chapter 8

Management of Mass Casualty Incidents

A mass casualty incident is defined as an incident overwhelming the available resources of the emergency medical service.

To avoid chaos, such an incident is managed according to Clausewitz's principles of order of time and space[56]. The time can be structured in three phases, initial, catch-up, and stabilisation[206]. The order of the space is shown in figure 8.3, page 91.

8.1 Initial Phase

The initial phase may also be termed 'chaos phase'. The major challenge is to establish orderly structures early, to allow proper incident management later and to enable reserves to integrate themselves into controlled incident management efforts[55]. At Ramstein, this 'chaos phase' was never overcome.

A member of the public or another emergency service alerts the fire/ambulance control. The control activates a predetermined response according to one of four Gefahrenabwehrstufe GAS incident response levels[184]:

GAS 1 — normal everyday work, no special means required, e.g. medical emergencies, road traffic accident with a small number of patients. Leadership by those involved, e.g. immediate care doctor, paramedic, and fire/rescue team leader

1. Do not treat patients — treatment of one patient will delay help for all

2. Short feedback to fire/ambulance control ("mass casualty incident caused by ..., incident progressing (e.g. fire)/static (e.g. coach accident), medical/ambulance incident officers required, more information soon") — allows control to activate means of predetermined attendance

3. Gain an overview. The team stays together, reports to other services, if already available. How many (major) casualties? Dangers of scene? Technical rescue/hazardous materials team etc required?

4. Detailed situation report to control: Approximate number of patients, number of patients with threatened vital functions, requirements for additional immediate care doctors, ALS ambulances, helicopters, hospital capacities, other services (e.g fire, rescue, hazardous materials)

5. Take over (initial) command — 'temporary medical/ambulance incident officers'. Determine site for casualty collection point. Structure casualty collection point (receiving/registration point, treatment area, casualty loading point)

6. Stop spontaneous transports — keep capacities of ambulances and hospitals for the most severely injured

7. Triage and treatment — triage first, then treatment of immediate (red) patients. Check need for priority treatment/transport

8. Give tasks to arriving emergency medical services. Formulate tasks clearly

9. Plan transport — patient/hospital/means of transport. Order transport for transport priority patients, inform control

10. Handover to medical/ambulance incident officers — situation, organization, transports up to now. Ask for new task

Table 8.1: Ten commandments for the first medical team

Based on an analysis of common mistakes, Th Uhr[255] developed these commandments to help the first arriving team to structure the scene of a major incident. A laminated card with these instructions can often be found in emergency medical service vehicles

GAS 2 — larger incident, just manageable with available means, e.g. road traffic accident with several casualties, or a hazardous materials incident with casualties. Reserves may be activated for area cover, e.g. firefighters/paramedics switch over from a water tender to an advanced life support ambulance, independent aid associations or ambulance service providers may be called, or mutual aid. Leadership by the first arriving immediate care doctor, paramedic, and fire officer ('bronze command')

GAS 3 — major incident, own resources not enough to cope, full activation of reserves required, e.g. train derailment, bus accident, terrorist bombing. Leadership by medical/ambulance/fire incident officers in TEL (technische Einsatzleitung, 'silver command)' with several sectors (EAL, Einsatzabschnittsleitung, 'bronze command')

GAS 4 — catastrophe, likely to overwhelm community resources, reserves, and regional trauma centres. Full command structures of DV100 incident management system ('gold command')

The incident response levels are used flexibly, depending on available assets (e.g. rural Peine county (Lower Saxony) with one immediate care doctor and three advanced life support ambulances at night will activate higher response levels far sooner than e.g. the city of Hamburg with two physician-staffed helicopters, eight ground-based immediate care doctors, and 74 advanced life support ambulances). The first team to arrive on the scene is responsible for activating back up and for creating some basic structures (table 8.1, page 86).

8.2   Catch-up Phase

A basic structure of the incident has already been established. Now the commanders and reserves arrive. The medical and ambulance incident officers take over command. A TEL (technische Einsatzleitung/'silver' command) is set up. Sectors with sector leaders (EAL — Einsatzabschnittsleitung) are formed. The scene is structured further (figure 8.3, page 91). An advanced medical

Entry

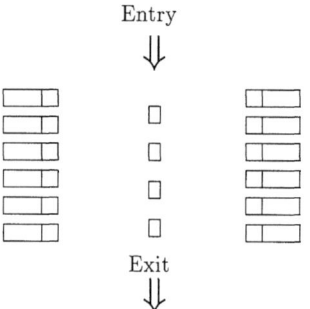

Exit

Figure 8.1: Casualty collection point

Two rows of stretchers, boxes of emergency equipment in the middle. Just outside the danger area, this is the place where the fire/rescue service hands over casualties to the emergency medical services. Showing a simple drawing like this to aiders, e.g. police or volunteer firemen, will enable them to help set up a casualty collection point.

post is established (figure 8.2, page 89). Further reserves are mobilised (aim: 1 immediate care doctor for 5 patients, one 'helper' for one patient). Patients are distributed to many different trauma centres.

8.2.1 Advanced medical post

Like in most European countries, the advanced medical post is the centerpiece of medical incident management[101, 192, 114]. The EAL (sector/'bronze' command) of the advanced medical post coordinates the activities in this area. It cooperates closely with the other sector commanders, especially the ones in charge of the ambulance waiting area and the helicopter landing field[186].
The advanced medical post is structured as a one way system[207, 208]: Patients enter via a triage/registration area. An immediate care doctor supported by several helpers triages the casualties. T1 immediate treatment (red) patients receive advanced lifesaving treatment (rapid sequence induction for airway management, ventilation, chest drains, control of haemorrhage, fluid resuscitation in the T1 area which usually consists of ≈ three mobile intensive care units/advanced life support ambulances and a tent as resuscitation rooms. Urgent priority transport (e.g. for surgical control of

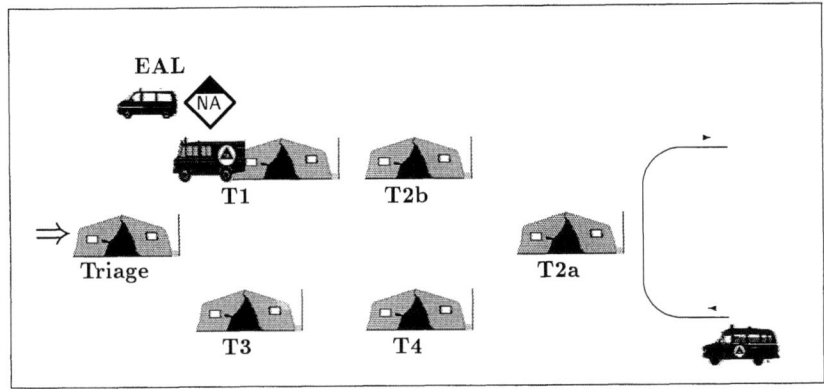

Figure 8.2: Advanced medical post

haemorrhage) may be required.

T2a patients (transport priority) are collected in a tent near the ambulance loading point. Oxygen can be supplied and intravenous access obtained while waiting for transport.

The T2b (stretcher cases, delayed transport) tent serves as a holding area, until enough ambulances are available.

T3 (green, walking wounded) casualties are collected in a tent. First aiders supervised by a paramedic or local general practitioner provide some basic care until transport.

T4 patients (expectant management) receive pain relief and spiritual care in a quiet area.

8.2.2 Triage

Triage is a dynamic, often repeated process. It is a medical task not normally delegated to paramedical staff. While in the initial phase a simple protocol-based method like START (simple triage and rapid treatment) is used, later triage is based on clinical judgement. Regular training courses, e.g. by the German Society for Disaster Medizine (DGKM — Deutsche Gesellschaft für Katastrophenmedizin) help to develop the necessary skills and judgement. Commonly used categories are:

T1 — immediate (red), treatment priority, casualties requiring interventions to restore or maintain vital functions

T2 — yellow, initially stable patients requiring skilled transport and hospital treatment. This category is subdivided into:

T2a — transport priority, casualties requiring urgent interventions in hospital, e.g. extremity fractures with neurovascular compromise

T2b — delayed transport, patients needing hospital treatment not endangered by some delay, e.g. uncomplicated limb fractures

T3 — minor injuries (green), no priority

T4 — hopeless under the circumstances (black or blue). The medical incident officer has to judge whether this category is necessary, or whether these patients should be treated as T1, immediate.

The injured are marked with triage tags. Two systems are in common use: Either the red cross card (cardboard, based on updated 2nd World War models, very cheap — can be used for exercises without much expense)[118, 197] or variants of the Swiss casualty handling system (plastic, modern, colour coded, expensive — rarely used for exercises)[176, 193, 115]. In the long run, probably the latter will prevail. It is also used in Austria and several eastern European states.

8.2.3   Dispersal

The casualties are distributed to many trauma centres to enable rapid treatment to the standards of individual medicine and to avoid overloading a few hospitals, while others stand by without receiving a single patient. Common bottlenecks in the hospitals are computed tomography and intensive care beds. Dispersal protects these resources. For efficient dispersal, large numbers of ambulances and helicopters are needed. The vehicles may have to do long journeys to distant trauma centres and are therefore not available for many repeat short round trips. Good communication with hospitals and ambulance controls becomes most important. Careful documentation of which patient went to which trauma

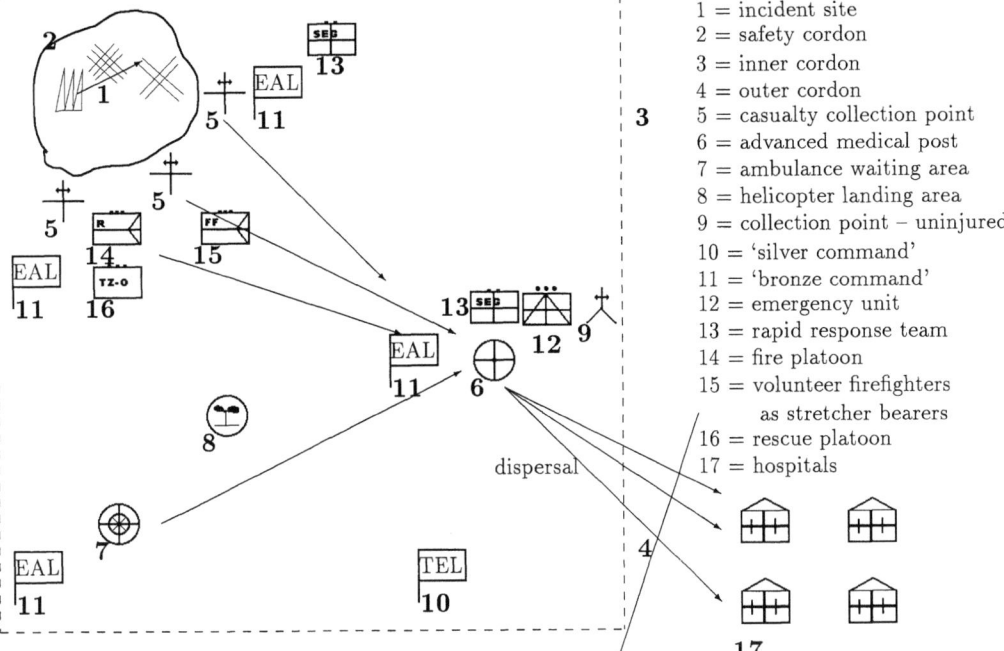

Figure 8.3: Order of space at major incidents

A TEL (10, 'silver command') with medical and ambulance incident officers is in charge of four 'bronze' sectors: Firefighting/rescue (1, with a fire and a rescue platoon), forward medical care/casualty collection points (5, with a rapid response team and stretcher bearers), advanced medical post (6)/collection point for the uninjured (9, with an emergency unit – see figure 3.8, page 34 and a rapid response team), and ambulance waiting area (7)/helicopter landing area (8)

centre by which means is essential to avoid overwhelming individual centres.

8.3   Stabilisation Phase

Now the means available correspond to the needs, there is at least one immediate care doctor for five casualties and one 'helper' for one patient. Individual standard emergency medicine has returned. Patients will be dispersed widely to often distant hospitals. The T3 walking wounded patients are transported to office-based doctors (e.g. general or orthopaedic surgeons, ophthalmologists, general practitioners) or hospital outpatient departments. The uninjured receive advice about counselling and are taken care of.

The aid personnel may be offered critical incident stress debriefing. Once released from the incident site, units will return to their bases, restock and repair equipment, preparing for the next callout. The incident officers complete their reports. Some days later, a debriefing is held. Issues and criticism can be discussed openly and lessons learned.

Chapter 9

Case Study: The Train Derailment at Eschede 1998

At 1059h on the 3rd of June 1998 a high speed InterCity Express train (travelling from Munich via Hanover to Hamburg) derailed at Eschede. The emergency services of a rural county were faced with the largest railway accident in the history of the Federal Republic of Germany. Some coaches hit a bridge which collapsed onto the wreckage, others folded one over the other. Eyewitnesses alerted the local volunteer fire brigade and the ambulance control of Celle County[214].

9.1 The Accident

This description is based on the symposium[127], other publications [227, 62, 125 202, 145, 89], and last not least on the experiences of doctors and other helpers whom I met.

9.1.1 Initial Phase

An advanced life support ambulance stationed in Eschede was the first emergency medical service team to reach the incident, followed by an immediate care doctor of Celle County General Hospital (level 2 trauma centre), and the other ALS ambulances of the county (ambulance service run jointly by the Red Cross and a private provider). A first impression was fed back to control who activated the county major incident plan. Basic life support ambulances of the county ambulance service and the independent providers (Order of Malta, private providers) and further trained immediate care doctors of the county hospital, including the designated medical incident officer, followed. Mutual aid was invoked, helicopters alerted (both the primary 'Christoph' air ambulances and intensive transfer helicopters), two emergency units (figure 3.8, page 34) of the civil defence/state disaster control (Celletown, Celle-county) called, and military support requested. Celle county did not have any rapid response teams relying on the emergency units instead. With all these units trying to find their way and attempting to make radio contact, the ambulance service radio channel got overloaded quickly. The fire service and civil defence channels failed as well as the mobile telephone network. The scene was divided into a western and eastern half by the wreckage. The only street crossing had been the collapsed bridge. Vehicles could not cross from one side to the other except at distant bridges. The site had to be structured accordingly. While the first immediate care doctor and his paramedic driver took command on one side, the other was soon handed to the team of the Christoph 4 air ambulance (Hanover medical school)[125]. Casualty collection points and ambulance waiting areas were established on either side. The order of 'transport stop' was given early. It worked well: Celle County hospital received twelve patients only during the whole day, most of them initially by spontaneous transports. The accident caused 91 people to die immediately. Of the 74 severely injured, five died on scene. 18 patients had minor injuries. The county medical incident officer arrived soon.

9.1.2 Catch-up Phase

The Technische Einsatzleitung (TEL, 'silver' command) was headed by the senior fire officer of the county. It was supported by the well equipped TEL unit of Hanover county. A Katastrophenschutzleitung (KatSL, 'gold' command) was established in the county hall. Advanced medical posts, each commanded by an experienced helicopter doctor, ambulance waiting areas and helicopter landing fields were set up on either side of the track. These structures were in place early and allowed the arriving mutual aid units, rapid response teams, the military, and other reserves to integrate without causing chaos. After assessment of the situation the medical incident officer decided that the triage category T4 (expectant management) should not be used. Within two hours over 80 immediate care doctors were present. Individual treatment to the standards of the regular emergency medical service became a realistic option. Patient dispersal to 23 level one and two trauma centres all over northern Germany ensured that no hospital had to deal with more than three to four patients[126]. The compound materials used to build the high speed train proved a major problem for the fire/rescue service. Heavy rescue units of the THW (Technisches Hilfswerk, technical aid association, a federal civil defence agency) were required.

9.1.3 Stabilisation Phase

After just 50 minutes the number of immediate care doctors and ambulance staff enabled the provision of individual medicine. Three hours after the event all regular professional ambulances were returned to their normal duties, the capacities of the rapid response teams and emergency units were sufficient. Only three patients needed secondary transfers. A large number of priests, social workers, and psychologists trained in critical incident stress management supported the helpers. A symposium was held five months later to learn from success and mistakes[127].

standards and measures	
Regular emergency services: Availability of emergency doctors, helicopters ALS, and BLS ambulances within 15, 30, and 60 min (radius of 10, 20, and 40 km (ground) or 50, 100, and 200 km(air))	1/2/33 helicopters: 4/4/9 ALS 6/11/94 BLS 11/4/89
rapid response teams within 20/40 km	$0/\approx 10$
state disaster units/ civil defence within 20/40 km	3/8
military/ other support within 60 min	stationed in county
standard: 1 doctor for 5 patients	achieved early
standard: 1 'helper' (from paramedic to civil defence aidman) for 1 patient	achieved early
qualification of aid personnel	skill mix
medical command structure: medical incident officer ambulance incident officer command support	well established yes yes Hanover County TEL
advanced medical post: team and equipment	emergency units and rapid response teams
trauma centers (level 1 − 3) within a distance of 30/60 minutes by ground/ by air	by air: level 1 1/7 level 2 by ground 2/15 by air 33/>50
burns beds within 60 minutes	not required

Table 9.1: Audit standards of structural quality

Data from 127, 75, 81

9.2 Lessons Learned

9.2.1 What worked well

— The DV100 incident management system proved itself. Order was established very early. This may be related to the familiarity of local emergency services with the DV100 system (Celle county got frequent brush fires). The 'new' staff functions S5 (media) and S6 (communications) were very useful given the media interest and the difficulties with radio communication[89].

— Reserves were activated rapidly and in sufficient numbers. Own reserves, including aid associations/independent providers not normally part of the county emergency medical service, were activated. The emergency units of the state disaster control and numerous rapid response teams brought quickly a large number of trained and disciplined helpers willing to work in a structured way. Generous helicopter support (34 helicopters) allowed the dispersal of the casualties with life-threatening injuries to trauma centres with available intensive care beds all over northern Germany. Military assets, including those of the British forces stationed in the county, were integrated well with civilian efforts.

— The initial breakdown of radio communications (the mobile phone networks were overloaded as well) was overcome soon by the TEL ('silver command'). The TEL unit from Hanover county (command bus, radio communications bus, two equipment vans) [154] proved invaluable.

— The rapid response teams and emergency units showed a high degree of skill and discipline. The skill-mix of off-duty professionals and volunteers, ranging from immediate care doctors and paramedics to civil defence aidmen seemed a recipe for success: Team members with lesser training were not left to 'get on with it', but assisted the more skilled, helped with documentation, served as runners and stretcher bearers, setting the fully trained members free for immediate patient care.

— A team of the British Army (stationed in the region) was well integrated into the medical and rescue efforts. This was partly due to the British commander's willingness to integrate the team into existing civilian command structures and partly due to the help of a German Army liaison officer who 'coordinated' the team's work[108]. The British commander's surprise that a German medical incident officer at an incident in Germany used German as the command language[62] illustrates the limits of help by NATO allies and the need for federal armed forces liaison officers.

— Psychosocial aftercare was well organised and received extra state funding for a long-term counselling centre[111].

9.2.2 Problems

— Recognition of the medical incident officer: 23 doctors wore turnout gear marked 'LNA' ('Leitender Notarzt'/medical incident officer)[126]. They held this function in their own counties. The medical incident officer should be recognizable easily, nobody else should look like this function.

— Communications broke down initially (see above).

— Some emergency units and rapid response teams deployed their vehicles individually, as soon as enough volunteers for one vehicle arrived. The vehicles of some teams arrived at different times and got allocated to different areas. The units did not work together as a team as they had trained to do. Such units should arrive as units and be deployed as units to increase their effectiveness[70].

— Railways: Initially some responders did ignore the electrical wires dangling around. In fact, they had been switched off within minutes, but the fire safety officer was informed with some delay only. Communications with the railway incident manager have been criticised, especially with regard to technical rescue.

— Access to the entrapped casualties and technical rescue proved extremely difficult owing to the compound materials of the high-speed train. A tunnel rescue train with both the required technical and medical equipment, staffed by the fire brigade and ambulance service of the town of Hildesheim was not called to the incident (on open track) for over one hour. It arrived too late to help in the rescue of live casualties[89]. The technical aid association, a federal civil defence agency, deployed its regional rescue platoons with heavy equipment.

— Some journalists hovered over the scene in a helicopter, endangering the starting and landing air ambulances (the airspace was closed to nonessential traffic rapidly)[145]. Others tried to get hold of spectacular pictures by sneaking through the cordons disguised

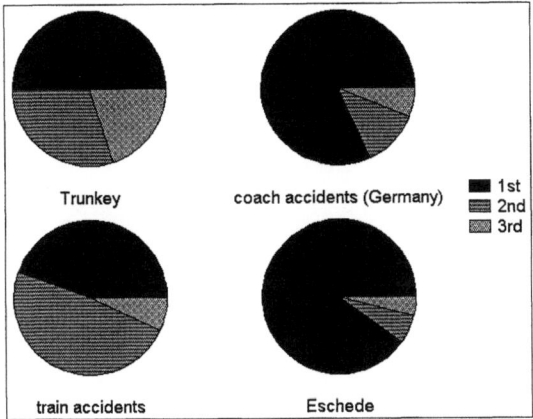

Figure 9.1: Trimodal distribution of death at Eschede

This incident was managed as successful as the coach accidents. A comparison with the average of many train accidents shows an excellent outcome

as priests or psychosocial care providers. Some ambulance crews got offered money to open the doors of their vehicles to allow photographers to take pictures of the casualties. Most journalists accepted their code of conduct and did not participate in such activities[251].

— Self-deployment of ambulances and rapid response teams made it difficult to keep an overview on the assets available. Clearly designated ambulance waiting areas helped to contain this problem.

9.3 Applying the Audit Tool

9.3.1 Structural Quality

Structural quality was high (table 9.1, page 96). Celle county did not have rapid response teams at this point. Mutual aid by the teams of neighbouring counties is available within a reasonable timeframe, as are two disaster control/civil defence emergency units. The county ambulance control was staffed by one person only. After the experience of this incident it was joined with the county fire control to an integrated fire/ambulance control.

standards and measures	
first team does not start treatment	did not start treatment
provides short feedback to control	yes
gains an overview	yes
establishes command & control	yes
first command: "transport stop" — no spontaneous, uncontrolled transports to hospitals	given early few (Celle County hospital received a total of 12 patients)
reserves: time for control to mobilize backup were mutual aid, rapid response teams, disaster units, civil defence, the military, and independent providers called early? not enough or too many reserves mobilized?	rapid yes, except for Hildesheim rescue train (called after 1h) adaequate
triage use of established categories initial, e.g. START flexible, adapted to situation or protocol-based? dynamic, repeated over-/undertriage	T4 not used no flexible yes individual medicine
stabilisation of 'immediate' patients before transport	yes
inappropriate procedures, e.g. CPR	—
handover to medical/ ambulance incident officers	yes
communication: breakdown of radio network?	initially, then controlled by TEL
advanced medical post established	early
ambulance waiting area	yes
no self-deployment of ambulances/ teams ('disaster tourism')	did happen
dispersal to different hospitals	to 23
number of secondary (hospital to hospital) transfers	3

Table 9.2: Audit standards of process quality

9.3.2 Process Quality

The first teams on scene set up structures very early on. This seems to be the key to success (table 9.2, page 100).

9.3.3 Outcome Quality

The outcome was remarkable (figure 9.1, page 99): The 91 immediate deaths attest to the force of the impact. Even though the mechanism of injury did cause severe injuries, only five patients died on scene after the arrival of the emergency medical services and one in an emergency department. Four late deaths in intensive care units compare favourably with the high number (68) of admissions to critical care .

The implementation of improvements in the three areas command & control, rapid mobilization of reserves, and incident management (structuring of scene, triage, and dispersal) made polytrauma a survivable disease even in a mass casualty incident.

Chapter 10

Conclusions

This text describes the German system for the medical management of major incidents. It may be helpful for those deploying to Germany.

The medical management of mass casualty incidents has changed markedly in the last 15 years. The two driving forces were:
The progress in prehospital emergency medicine, especially trauma care where 'treat & run' has superseded 'stay & stabilise'.
The transformation of war leading to a transformation of civil defence. For the thousand bomber raids of the 2nd world war or the nuclear stalemate civil defence preparations could be kept separate from peacetime emergency services. Todays 'low-intensity conflicts' require a close integration of all available emergency services. Germany has managed to successfully integrate its civil defence assets into peacetime major incident preparations. Major incidents can be caused accidentally, by the risks of our technologies, or deliberately, by fanatical warriors/terrorists. The result is the same: A mass casualty incident.
Major incident management can be audited using the methods of total quality management. The trimodal distribution of trauma death is developed as a tool for the audit of outcomes. It can be applied to any emergency system. The trimodal distribution of death shows the German major incident trauma care in a particularly bright light. It also affords insights into the limitations of

paramedic-only systems.

The much beloved 'freedom of speech', open, and often very frank discussions, allowed the German emergency services to improve their major incident management. Only by openly addressing problems and mistakes can lessons be learned.

The main changes implemented were: A strengthened system of command and control, based on the DV100 incident management system, and highly trained medical and ambulance incident officers.

A systematic way to receive reinforcements and activate reserves: Own resources, mutual aid, helicopters, rapid response teams, disaster control/civil defence, and military support, all integrated easily in one single command system (DV100).

Mass casualty incident management based on the three principles of structuring the scene early, triage, and dispersal with the aim of restoring individual patient care as soon as possible.

The two case studies of Ramstein 1988, and Eschede 1998 illustrate the difference these improvements made.

Many of these improvements could easily be transferred to other countries with different emergency systems.

The helicopter emergency medical service already is an export hit: Many countries use this model, often even painting their helicopters yellow, using the MBB Bo105 CBS, or even let their HEMS crew members wear orange German-style overalls.

The rapid response teams can by now be found in some other European countries, e.g. Austria or the Netherlands[99].

Other elements of the system might be useful abroad as well.

Abbreviations

A&E	accident and emergency
ADAC	Allgemeiner Deutscher Automobilclub
	German automobile association
ALS	advanced life support
ASB	Arbeiter-Samariter-Bund
	Workers' Samaritans aid organisation
ATLS	advanced trauma life support
ATrKw	Arzttruppkraftwagen
	medical squad vehicle
BLEVE	boiling liquid expanding vapour explosion
BLS	basic life support
BRK	Bayerisches Rotes Kreuz
	Bavarian Red Cross
CCU	coronary/cardiac care unit
CPR	cardiopulmonary resuscitation
DIN	Deutsches Institut für Normung
	German norm
DRF	Deutsche Rettungsflugwacht
	air rescue charity
DRK	Deutsches Rotes Kreuz
	German Red Cross
DV100	Dienstvorschrift 100
	German incident management system
EAL	Einsatzabschnittsleitung
	'bronze' command
ECG	electrocardiography
EMS	emergency medical service

EMT-B	emergency medical technician – basic
EMT-I	emergency medical technician – intermediate
EN	European norm
GAS	Gefahren-Abwehrstufe
	incident response level
HEMS	helicopter emergency medical service
HVB	Hauptverwaltungsbeamter
	senior administratve officer
	head of 'gold' command
IFA	Internationale Flug-Ambulanz
	air rescue charity
ITU	intensive treatment unit
iv	intravenous
JUH	Johanniter Unfall-Hilfe
	St John Ambulance
KatS	Katastrophenschutz
	disaster control
KatSL	Katastrophenschutzleitung
	'gold' command
KrLKW	Krankenlastkraftwagen
	auxiliary lorry ambulance
KTW	Krankentransportwagen
	BLS ambulance
LARMC	Landstuhl Army Regional Medical Center
LNA	Leitender Notarzt
	medical incident officer
LSHD	Luftschutzhilfsdienst
	air raid protection service
MHD	Malteser Hilfsdienst
	Order of Malta ambulance service
NA	Notarzt
	immediate care doctor
NACA	National Advisory Comittee on Aeronautics
	injury severity score

NAW	Notarztwagen
	mobile intensive care unit
NBC	nuclear/biological/chemical
NCO	non-commissioned officer
NEF	Notarzteinsatzfahrzeug
	immediate care doctor's speed intervention vehicle
ÖEL	Örtliche Einsatzleitung
	'silver' command
OrgL	Organisatorischer Leiter
	ambulance incident officer
PALS	paediatric advanced life support
RTH	Rettungstransporthubschrauber
	ambulance helicopter
RTS	Revised Trauma Score
RTW	Rettungstransportwagen
	ALS ambulance
SanGrKw	Sanitätsgruppenkraftwagen
	first aid section van
SAR	search & rescue
SEG	Schnell- or Sonder- Einsatzgruppe
	rapid response team
START	simple triage and rapid treatment
TEL	Technische Einsatzleitung
	'silver' command
THW	Technisches Hilfswerk
	technical aid association
	a federal civil defence agency
TRISS	Trauma Research Injury Severity Score
USAFE	US Air Force Europe
ZS	Zivilschutz
	civil defence

Bibliography

[1] V Aburel, L Visa, and D Grigorescu. The 1979 fire disaster (93 casualties) in brasov (romania) — the importance of rapid transport and unitary treatment in a hospital. *Ann Medit Burns Club*, 7(1):30 – 35, March 1994.

[2] Akademie für Notfallplanung und Zivilschutz im Bundesamt für Zivilschutz. Fort- und Weiterbildung an der AkNZ: Ärzte im Zivil- und Katastrophenschutz. *SEG – Zeitschrift für Schnell-Einsatz-Gruppen und erweiterten Rettungsdienst*, 5(2):67 – 68, 1998.

[3] anonymous. Moorgate tube train disaster. *Br Med J*, 3:727 – 731, 27 September 1975.

[4] anonymous. Reisebus überschlug sich — zwölf Notärzte im Einsatz. *Rettungs-Magazin*, 1(3):15, 1996.

[5] anonymous. Interregio kollidierte mit entgleistem Intercity. *Rettungs-Magazin*, 4(3):16, 1999.

[6] anonymous, editor. *Notruf 112. Feuerwehren im Einsatz*, volume 18. EFB, Erlensee, 1999.

[7] anonymous. Verteilung ist Ländersache. "Platzhalter" zur Vermeidung von Lücken im Fahrzeugbestand des Katastrophenschutzes. *Bevölkerungsschutz — Magazin für Zivil- und Katastrophenschutz*, (1):25, 1999.

[8] anonymous. 18 killed in south african train crash. http://www.ananova.com/news/story/sm_513940.html, accessed 30/07/2003 2000.

[9] anonymous. Fifteen injured in train collision. http://www.ananova.com/news/story/sm_153218.html, accessed 30/07/2003 2000.

[10] anonymous. One killed in head-on train collision. http://www.ananova.com/news/story/sm_153240.html, accessed 30/07/2003 2000.

[11] anonymous. Sanitäts- und Betreuungsdienst: Niedersachsen. *SEG – Zeitschrift für Schnell-Einsatz-Gruppen und erweiterten Rettungsdienst*, 7(5):210 – 211, 2000.

[12] anonymous. Schüler stritten sich — Bus prallt gegen Baum. *Rettungs-Magazin*, 5(2):14, 2000.

[13] anonymous. Death toll rises to 22 in south african train crash. http://www.ananova.com/news/story/sm_514439.html, accessed 30/07/2003 2002.

[14] anonymous. Potters bar train crash claims seventh victim. http://www.ananova.com/news/story/sm_585581.html, accessed 30/07/2003 2002.

[15] anonymous. Six dead and 100 injured as trains collide. http://www.ananova.com/news/story/sm_513780.html, accessed 30/07/2003 2002.

[16] anonymous. Sixth person dies after crash. http://www.ananova.com/news/story/sm_585440.html, accessed 30/07/2003 2002.

[17] anonymous. Surgeons battling to save lives of three crash victims. http://www.ananova.com/news/story/sm_585501.html, accessed 30/07/2003 2002.

[18] anonymous. Train crash in portugal kills five, injures seven. http://www.ananova.com/news/story/sm_560206.html, accessed 30/07/2003 2002.

[19] anonymous. Two dead in california train crash. http://www.ananova.com/news/story/sm_573680.html, accessed 30/07/2003 2002.

[20] anonymous. Witness tells of train horror. http://www.ananova.com/news/story/sm_585435.html, accessed 30/07/2003 2002.

[21] anonymous. 300 Helfer waren im Einsatz. http://www.feuerwehrmagazin.de/seiten/data/artikel/news.asp?id=2692, accessed 04/07/2003 2003.

[22] Arbeitsgemeinschaft in Norddeutschland tätiger Notärzte e.V. Therapieleitlinien für die Notfallmedizin. Braunschweig, 2000.

[23] Arbeitsgemeinschaft Notärzte NRW. Studie der AGNNW zur Strukturqualität. http://agnnw.de/2002/web/agnnw_empfehlungen_Q-M.html, accessed 1/8/2003, 2002.

[24] Arbeitskreis V. Neue Strategie zum Bevölkerungsschutz. Beschluss der Innenministerkonferenz. *Bevölkerungsschutz — Magazin für Zivil- und Katastrophenschutz*, (3):3 – 5, 2002.

[25] G Arturson. The los alfaques disaster: a boiling-liquid expanding-vapour explosion. *Burns*, 7(3):233 – 251, 1981.

[26] Ärztekammer Sachsen-Anhalt. Richtlinie zur Erteilung des Fachkundenachweises "Leitender Notarzt" in Sachsen-Anhalt, 1995.

[27] J Bahr. Breitenausbildung in Herz-Lungen-Wiederbelebung (HLW) - Ist eine Wirksamkeit erkennbar? In Weidringer et al. [264], pages 14 – 24.

[28] TL Barclay. Mass casualties. In JAD Settle, editor, *Principles and Practice of Burns Management*, chapter 4, pages 51 – 57. Churchill Livingstone, New York, 1996.

[29] R Bardua. "Mendiger CH 53–Modell". Ein Beispiel zivil–militärischer Zusammenarbeit. *Wehrmedizinische Monatsschrift*, (11):356 – 358, 1993.

[30] C Barnett. *The Lost Victory. British Dreams, British Realities 1945 – 1950*. Pan, London, 1996.

[31] S Beck. SEG'en im Südwesten. *SEG – Magazin für Schnelleinsatzgruppen*, 1(5):193 – 195, 1994.

[32] S Beck. MANV in Thüringen. *SEG – Zeitschrift für Schnell-Einsatz-Gruppen und erweiterten Rettungsdienst*, 7(2):82 – 83, 2000.

[33] A Biehle, editor. *Das Flugunglück von Ramstein am 28. August 1988: Beschlußempfehlung und Bericht des Verteidigungsausschusses als Untersuchungsausschuß; Beratung und Beschluß des Deutschen Bundestages*, volume 6/89 of *Zur Sache. Themen parlamentarischer Beratung*. Deutscher Bundestag, Referat Öffentlichkeitsarbeit, Bonn, 1989.

[34] W Birkholz. Interaktionen zwischen Rettungsdienst und Katastrophenschutz. Kritische Analyse und Lösungsmöglichkeiten. *SEG – Magazin für Schnelleinsatzgruppen*, 2(2):54 – 59, 1995.

[35] W Birkholz. Katastrophenschutz und Rettungsdienst. Sind getrennte Strukturen noch zeitgemäß? *SEG – Magazin für Schnelleinsatzgruppen*, 2(1):6 – 10, 1995.

[36] J Bittger. *Großunfälle und Katastrophen. Einsatztaktik und -organisation*. Schattauer, Stuttgart, 1996.

[37] I Blanck. Reanimation nach Wohnungsbrand. *Rettungs-Magazin*, 6(5):46 – 47, 2001.

[38] GV Bochicchio, O Ilahi, M Joshi, K Bochicchio, and TM Scalea. Endotracheal intubation in the field does not improve outcome in trauma patients who present without an acutely lethal traumatic brain injury. *J Trauma*, 54(2):307 – 311, Feb 2003.

[39] KH Bock, W Breschinski, and G Hölldobler. SAR: Rettungsdienst-Einrichtungen der Bundeswehr. *SEG – Magazin für Schnelleinsatzgruppen*, 3(4):206 – 207, 1996.

[40] S Bockting. *Feuerwehren im Ruhrgebiet.* EFB, Erlensee, 2000.

[41] P Buchner. "Si vis pacem" — oder: Den Zivilschutz gibt es noch. *SEG – Zeitschrift für Schnell-Einsatz-Gruppen und erweiterten Rettungsdienst*, 5:198 –199, 5 1998.

[42] Bundesamt für zivilen Bevölkerungsschutz. LSHD-DV 301, vorläufige Dienstvorschrift: Die LS-Sanitätsbereitschaft. Bad Godesberg, 1965.

[43] Bundesamt für Zivilschutz, Bonn. *STAN-Nr. 041. Sanitätszug*, 1984.

[44] Bundesärztekammer. Empfehlungen der Bundesärztekammer zur Fortbildung zum "Leitenden Notarzt". *Deutsches Ärzteblatt*, 85(8):A454 – A456, 25 February 1988.

[45] Bundesverwaltungsamt, Zentralstelle für Zivilschutz, Bonn. *Der ABC-Erkundungskraftwagen (ABC-ErkKW). Eine technische Kurzbeschreibung*, 2000.

[46] Bundesverwaltungsamt, Zentralstelle für Zivilschutz, Referat V A 2, Bonn. *Typenblatt Arzttrupp-Kraftwagen, Fahrzeugtyp DB-Kastenwagen, Typ L 407D/35.*

[47] Bundesverwaltungsamt, Zentralstelle für Zivilschutz, Referat V A 2, Bonn. *Typenblatt Arzttrupp-Kraftwagen, Fahrzeugtyp Ducato 14, Typ 290.*

[48] Bundesverwaltungsamt, Zentralstelle für Zivilschutz, Referat V A 2, Bonn. *Typenblatt Krankentransportwagen, Fahrzeugtyp FT130 / 82 E 4.*

[49] Bundesverwaltungsamt, Zentralstelle für Zivilschutz, Referat V A 2, Bonn. *Typenblatt Krankentransportwagen, Fahrzeugtyp FT 100L / VIL.*

[50] Bundesverwaltungsamt, Zentralstelle für Zivilschutz, Referat V A 2, Bonn. *Typenblatt Krankentransportwagen, Fahrzeugtyp FT 150 CL, Typ EAL.*

[51] Bundesverwaltungsamt, Zentralstelle für Zivilschutz, Referat V A 2, Bonn. *Typenblatt Krankentransportwagen, Fahrzeugtyp 313 CDI/35 Sprinter.*

[52] Bundesverwaltungsamt, Zentralstelle für Zivilschutz, Referat V A 2, Bonn. *Typenblatt Sanitätsgruppen-Kraftwagen, Fahrzeugtyp FT 100 / VLS.*

[53] Bundesverwaltungsamt, Zentralstelle für Zivilschutz, Referat V A 2, Bonn. *Typenblatt Sanitätsgruppen-Kraftwagen, Fahrzeugtyp FT 100 CL / EDS.*

[54] G Carloff. Luftrettungsdienst. In Crespin and Peter [65], chapter 12, pages 232 – 239.

[55] U Cimolino, MHaisch, T Lembeck, and S Taylor. *Technische Hilfeleistung bei Busunfällen.* Einsatzpraxis. ecomed Sicherheit, Landsberg, 2001.

[56] C von Clausewitz. *Vom Kriege.* Propyläen Taschenbuch. Ullstein, Berlin, 2nd edition, 1999.

[57] B Coellen and M Tiedt. Die SEG des landeseigenen Katastrophenschutzes im Land Brandenburg. In *Referateband Fachtagung Schnelleinsatzgruppen in Potsdam, 19. 06. 1993*, pages 14 – 25, Köln, 1994. Arbeiter–Samariter– Bund Deutschland e.V.

[58] B Coellen and M Tiedt. Die SEG'en im Land Brandenburg. *SEG – Magazin für Schnelleinsatzgruppen*, 1(2):73 – 74, 1994.

[59] B Coellen and M Tiedt. Die Sonder-Einsatz-Gruppen im Land Brandenburg. In Mitschke and Peter [187], chapter 11.8, pages 337 – 344.

[60] Committee on Trauma, American College of Surgeons, editor. *Advanced Trauma Life Support for Doctors. Student Course Manual.* American College of Surgeons, Chicago, IL, 6th edition, 1997.

[61] A Cooper, C DiScala, G Foltin, M Tunik, D Markenson, and C Welborn. Prehospital endotracheal intubation for severe head injury in children: a reappraisal. *Semin Pediatr Surg*, 10(1):3 – 6, Feb 2001.

[62] R Cordell. The eschede rail crash, germany, 3 june 1998: a british observer's report. *Pre-hospital Immediate Care*, 4(4):196 – 200, December 2000.

[63] UB Crespin. Das Bombenattentat von Euskirchen. Einsatzmanagement und –nachbereitung. *SEG – Magazin für Schnelleinsatzgruppen*, 1(3):112 – 117, 1994.

[64] UB Crespin and G Neff, editors. *Handbuch der Sichtung.* Themenschwerpunkt. Stumpf & Kossendey, Edewecht, 2000.

[65] UB Crespin and H Peter, editors. *Handbuch für Organisatorische Leiter.* Stumpf & Kossendey, Edewecht, 1996.

[66] M van Creveld. *The Transformation of War.* Free Press, New York, 1991.

[67] DP Davis, DB Hoyt, M Ochs, D Fortlage, T Holbrook, LK Marshall, and P Rosen. The effect of paramedic rapid sequence intubation on outcome in patients with severe traumatic brain injury. *J Trauma*, 54(3):444 – 453, Mar 2003.

[68] D Demetriades, L Chan, E Cornwell, H Belzberg, TV Berne, J Asensio, D Chan, M Eckstein, and K Alo. Paramedic vs private transportation of trauma patients. effect on outcome. *Arch Surg*, 131(2):133 – 138, Feb 1996.

[69] Deutscher Bundestag. Protokoll der 175. Sitzung – 11. Wahlperiode, Bonn, Mittwoch, 15. November 1989.

[70] Deutsches Rotes Kreuz, Landesverband Niedersachsen. Das Zugunglück in Eschede. Nachbereitung des Einsatzes, 1998.

[71] M Dietrich. Schwebebahn-Absturz in Wuppertal. *112 – Magazin der Feuerwehr*, 24(7):386 – 390, July 1999.

[72] M Dörmann. SEG-Regionalstruktur Nordrhein-Westfalen. *SEG – Magazin für Schnelleinsatzgruppen*, 2(2):72 – 81, 1995.

[73] MR Dörmann. Fortbildung für Leitende Notärzte. *SEG – Zeitschrift für Schnell-Einsatz-Gruppen und erweiterten Rettungsdienst*, 5(1):27 – 29, 1998.

[74] MR Dörmann. LNA Fortbildung: Flugunfälle. *SEG – Zeitschrift für Schnell-Einsatz-Gruppen und erweiterten Rettungsdienst*, 5(3):140 – 141, 1998.

[75] MR Dörmann. *Taschenkalender 1999*. Stumpf & Kossendey, Edewecht, 1998.

[76] R Ebhart, M Wilczek, and U Stiaßny. 3 Stunden eingeklemmt. *Rettungs-Magazin*, 7(4):42 – 44, 2002.

[77] M Eichner. Neues Glied in der Rettungskette? Freiwillige Feuerwehren als First-Responder-Einheit. *Rettungs-Magazin*, 1(2):84 – 87, März/April 1996.

[78] A Ekkernkamp and A David. Fortbildung zum Leitenden Notarzt — wer nimmt die Möglichkeit wahr? In Hierholzer and Böhm [116], pages 15 – 17.

[79] A Elklit. The aftermath of an industrial disaster. *Acta Psychiatrica Scandinavica*, 392(supplementum):1 – 25, 1997.

[80] K Ellinger and M Quiniel. Das Ramstein Unglück. *Notarzt*, 5:68, 1989.

[81] HA Emminger. *Klink, die Klinikdatenbank version 1.0*. Compare, Frankfurt, 1996.

[82] GH Engelhardt, editor. *Rettungsdienst in Europa. Referateband 16. Bundeskongress Rettungsdienst Aachen 1996*, Edewecht, 1996. Stumpf & Kossendey.

[83] GH Engelhardt, editor. *Der Rettungsdienst vor neuen Herausforderungen. Medizin, Ausbildung, Organisation. Referateband 18. Bundeskongreß Rettungsdienst Bremen 1998*, Edewecht, 1998. Stumpf & Kossendey.

[84] K Enke, M Wiethe, and M Homann. Vielseitig einsetzbar. SEG Hannover der JUH RV Nds. Mitte. *SEG – Zeitschrift für Schnell-Einsatz-Gruppen und erweiterten Rettungsdienst*, 7(2):77 – 79, 2000.

[85] DV Feliciano, GV Anderson, GS Rozycki, WL Ingram, JP Ansley andN Narnias, JP Salomone, and JD Cantwell. Management of casualties from the bombing at the centennial olympics. *Am J Surg*, 178:538 – 543, December 1998.

[86] B Fertig, editor. *Strategien gegen den plötzlichen Herztod*. Stumpf & Kossendey, Edewecht, 3 edition, 1997.

[87] M Folwaczny. Schwarzer Freitag. *Rettungs-Magazin*, 5(5):73, 2000.

[88] G Forty. *Land Warfare. The Encyclopedia of 20th Century Conflict*. Arms and Armour Press, London, 1997.

[89] L Franke. Eschede: Schweres ICE-Unglück. In anonymous [6], pages 6 – 14.

[90] J Fries. 11. Mainzer Fortbildungskurs LNA: Drei Großübungen vermitteln Praxiswissen. *SEG – Zeitschrift für Schnell-Einsatz-Gruppen und erweiterten Rettungsdienst*, 8(1):39 – 41, 2001.

[91] AH Fritzsche. 17 Tote bei Bahn-Unglück. *Feuerwehr-Magazin*, 7(5):30 – 34, May 1990.

[92] AH Fritzsche. SEG — Das Modell Rheinland-Pfalz: Grand mit Vieren. *Rettungs-Magazin*, 3(3):18 – 28, 1998.

[93] AH Fritzsche. Leipziger Allerlei. *Rettungs-Magazin*, 4(1):18 – 28, 1999.

[94] G Fröhlich. "Die Welt nachdenklich betrachten". Sicherheitspolitische Rahmenbedingungen für die Notfallplanung in Europa. *Bevölkerungsschutz — Magazin für Zivil- und Katastrophenschutz*, (3):3 – 6, 1999.

[95] ER Frykberg, JJ Tepas, and RH Alexander. The 1983 beirut airport terrorist bombing. injury patterns and implications for disaster management. *American Surgeon*, 55(3):134 – 141, 1989.

[96] M Geddert. Atemschutzgeräteträger in SEG'en. *SEG – Magazin für Schnelleinsatzgruppen*, 2(1):11 – 13, 1995.

[97] M Gihl. *Rettungsfahrzeuge. Von der Krankenkutsche zum Notarztwagen.* Edition Feuerwehr. W Kohlhammer, Stuttgart, 1986.

[98] PA Gomez Morell, F Escudero Naif, R Palao Domenech, E Sospedra Carol, and JA Bañuelos Roda. Burns caused by the terrorist bombing of the department store hipercor in barcelona. part i. *Burns,* 16(6):423 – 425, 1990.

[99] T Gras. Schnell–Einsatz–Gruppen in Amsterdam. *SEG – Magazin für Schnelleinsatzgruppen,* 1(1):6 – 11, 1994.

[100] F Grell. Verletzten-Leitkonzept für Großunfälle mit MANV. *SEG – Magazin für Schnelleinsatzgruppen,* 2(3):121 – 123, 1995.

[101] JL Guinaud and C Boyer. Advanced Medical post: Front medical collecting area or front triage area. In J de Boer and M Dubouloz, editors, *Handbook of Disaster Medicine: Emergency medicine in mass casualty situations,* chapter 7, pages 311 – 321. International Society of Disaster Medicine/Van der Wees, Utrecht, 2000.

[102] M Gutzmann. LS-Sanitätsdienst. In Koczy [148], pages 63 – 70.

[103] J Habers. *Vorbereitung der Einsatztaktik für den Großschadensfall im Organisationsbereich zwischen Rettungsdienst und Katastrophenschutz. Vergleichende Untersuchung aus notärztlicher Sicht.* MD thesis, Medizinische Fakultät der Rheinisch-Westfälischen Technischen Hochschule Aachen, Aachen, 1992.

[104] J Habers. KatS–Sanitätshelfer als Einsatzreserve. Zusätzliche Ausbildung für sinnvollen Einsatz im erweiterten Rettungsdienst. *SEG – Magazin für Schnelleinsatzgruppen,* 1(4):141 – 143, 1994.

[105] J Habers. Krankenhäuser. In Crespin and Peter [65], chapter 11, pages 212 – 231.

[106] J Habers. SEG-Verbandplatz: Zentrale Versorgungseinrichtung beim Massenanfall von Verletzten. In Engelhardt [82], pages 280 – 287.

[107] E Hampe. *Der Zivile Luftschutz im Zweiten Weltkrieg. Dokumentation und Erfahrungsberichte über Aufbau und Einsatz.* Bernhard & Graefe Verlag für Wehrwesen, Frankfurt/Main, 1963.

[108] HH Heidmann. Einsatz Bundeswehr. In Hüls and Oestern [127], chapter 2.3, pages 85 – 90.

[109] M Heimann, M Schnabel, and D Beetz. Schweres Zugunglück bei Neustadt. In anonymous [6], pages 80 – 86.

116

[110] HH Hellweg and B Domres. Definierte Materialausstattung einer SEG — machbar oder Fiktion? *SEG – Magazin für Schnelleinsatzgruppen*, 3(3):150 – 153, 1996.

[111] J Helmerichs. Einsatznachsorge beim ICE-Unglück in Eschede. In Hüls and Oestern [127], chapter 4.1, pages 119 – 124.

[112] J Herlitz, J Bahr, M Fischer, M Kuisma, K Lexow, and G Thorgeirson. Resuscitation in europe: A tale of five european regions. *Resuscitation*, 41(2):121 – 131, 1999.

[113] A Hermens. Die "Grünen Jacken". Sonder-Einsatz-Gruppen Betreuung in Brandenburg. *SEG – Magazin für Schnelleinsatzgruppen*, 4(2):76 – 77, 1997.

[114] A Hernando Lorenzo, FJ Estella Lana, and N Perales R de Viguri. La alerta y alarma. sistemas de comunicaciones. puesto de mando avanzado. In C Alvarez Leiva, V Chuliá Campos, and A Hernando Lorenzo, editors, *Manual de asistencia sanitaria en las catástrofes*, chapter 8, pages 83 – 101. Editorial Libro del Año, Madrid, 1992.

[115] B Hersche. PLS — Patientenleitsystem. In Crespin and Neff [64], chapter 3.5.3, pages 192 – 200.

[116] G Hierholzer and HJ Böhm, editors. *Der Massenunfall in Verkehr und Arbeitswelt*, volume 8 of *Traumatologie aktuell*. G Thieme, Stuttgart, 1992.

[117] F Hitz. Einsatzerfahrung: Flughafen Düsseldorf. In Peter and Maurer [204], chapter 4, pages 57 – 78.

[118] F Hitz and J von der Heidt. 14mal ge-MANV-t: Seminar "Massenanfall von Verletzten oder Erkrankten" der BF Düsseldorf. *SEG – Magazin für Schnelleinsatzgruppen*, 6(3):127 – 129, 1999.

[119] TJ Hodgetts and K Mackway-Jones, editors. *Major Incident Medical Management and Support. The Practical Approach at the Scene*. BMJ Books, London, 2nd edition, 2002.

[120] H Hofmann, S Niemann, and J Michel. Einsatz von FW, Rettungsdienst und SEG: Wohnhausbrand. *SEG – Zeitschrift für Schnell-Einsatz-Gruppen und erweiterten Rettungsdienst*, 5(3):118 – 121, 1998.

[121] A Hofmeister and MR Schütz. Ortsfeuerwehr Lemförde: Erste-Hilfe-Team "Löschen und mehr". *SEG – Zeitschrift für Schnell-Einsatz-Gruppen und erweiterten Rettungsdienst*, 7(1):29 –30, 2000.

[122] DE Hogan, JF Waeckerle, DJ Dire, and SR Lillibridge. Emergency department impact of the oklahoma city terrorist bombing. *Ann Emerg Med*, 34(2):160 – 167, August 1999.

[123] J Hornig. Zivilschutzhubschrauber im Rettungsdienst. *Bevölkerungsschutz — Magazin für Zivil- und Katastrophenschutz*, (3):8 – 10, 1998.

[124] PG Hoving. Der große Knall. Explosionsunglück in Enschede (Niederlande). *Rettungs-Magazin*, 5(5):18 – 22, 2000.

[125] V Hubrich. Bericht aus Sicht des Rettungsassistenten des Rettungshubschraubers Christoph 4. In Engelhardt [83], pages 484 – 486.

[126] E Hüls. Einsatz Rettungsdienst. In Hüls and Oestern [127], chapter 1.1, pages 3 – 29.

[127] E Hüls and HJ Oestern, editors. *Die ICE-Katastrophe von Eschede. Erfahrungen und Lehren. Eine Interdisziplinäre Analyse*. Springer, Berlin, 1999.

[128] E Iliopoulou, A Lochaitis, E Komninakis, L Poulikakos, S Asfour, S Chalkitis, and C Tzortzis. Mass disasters in greece. *Ann Medit Burns Club*, 7(1):36 – 39, March 1994.

[129] T Immenroth. First Responder von der Schulbank. *Rettungs-Magazin*, 6(5):30 – 34, 2001.

[130] DM Jackson. Causes and classification of accident burns and assessment of the patient. In C Wood, editor, *Accident and Emergency Burns: Lessons from the Bradford Disaster*, number 3 in Round Table Series, pages –. Royal Society of Medicine Services, London, 1986.

[131] H Jatzko and MR Dörmann. Psychologische Betreuung nach einem Busunglück. *SEG – Zeitschrift für Schnell-Einsatz-Gruppen und erweiterten Rettungsdienst*, 5(5):224, 1998.

[132] H Jatzko, S Jatzko, and H Seidlitz. *Das durchstoßene Herz: Ramstein 1988. Beispiel einer Katastrophen-Nachsorge*. Stumpf & Kossendey, Edewecht, 1995.

[133] W Jendsch. Benebelt. Massenkarambolage auf der A8 bei Ulm. *Rettungs-Magazin*, 4(3):66 – 71, 1999.

[134] W Jendsch. Vom Vorbild zum Modell. Die Einsatzfahrzeuge des Katastrophenschutzes. Heute: Krankentransportwagen (KTW) des LSHD. *Bevölkerungsschutz — Magazin für Zivil- und Katastrophenschutz*, (2):59, 2001.

[135] W Jendsch. Bus hängt am Steilhang. *Rettungs-Magazin*, 7(2):40 – 43, 2002.

[136] W Jendsch. Crash vor Piste 28. Crossair-Absturz bei Bassersdorf/Schweiz. *Rettungs-Magazin*, 7(3):28 – 30, 2002.

[137] FH Jimenez-Hernandez, E Lliro Blasco, R Leiva Oliva, JC Caicedo Caicedo, and JA Bañuelos Roda. Burns caused by the terrorist bombing of the department store hipercor in barcelona. part 2. *Burns*, 16(6):426 – 431, 1990.

[138] M Job. *Air Disaster*, volume 1. Aerospace Publications, Weston Creek, 1994.

[139] M Job. *Air Disaster*, volume 2. Aerospace Publications, Weston Creek, 1996.

[140] M Job. *Air Disaster*, volume 3. Aerospace Publications, Weston Creek, 1998.

[141] U Kämmerer and HG Winschermann. "Drama begann um 10.00 Uhr ..." Fallbeispiel: Verbrennungstrauma. *Rettungsdienst*, 18(9):717 –718, 1995.

[142] E Katz, B Ofek, J Adler, HB Abramowitz, and MM Krausz. Primary blast injury after a bomb explosion in a civilian bus. *Ann Surg*, 209(4):484 – 488, 1989.

[143] U Kippnich. Übung der hessischen Schnelleinsatzzüge '94. Eine Veranstaltung, die ihresgleichen sucht. *SEG – Magazin für Schnelleinsatzgruppen*, 1(5):212 – 215, 1994.

[144] U Kippnich. Das Sekretariat des Einsatzleiters. *Rettungs-Magazin*, 8(3):58 – 60, 2003.

[145] F Knobling. Bericht aus der Sicht des ersteintreffenden Rettungsteams. In Engelhardt [83], pages 487 – 491.

[146] H Knoche. Der Sanitätsdienst der Bundeswehr. In Crespin and Peter [65], chapter 13, pages 240 – 263.

[147] H Knoche. Zivil-militärische Zusammenarbeit in Nordrhein-Westfalen. Konzeptionelle Überlegungen zu einem Modellprojekt im Gesundheitswesen. *SEG – Magazin für Schnelleinsatzgruppen*, 3(4):222 – 225, 1996.

[148] A Koczy, editor. *Der Luftschutzhilfsdienst. Allgemeiner Leitfaden für Helfer*. Number 1 in Schriftenreihe Ziviler Bevölkerungsschutz. Deutscher Fachschriften-Verlag Braun, Wiesbaden-Dotzheim, 1960.

[149] T Kossmann and O Trentz. Flugschauunglück Ramstein 1988. Erfahrungsbericht eines betroffenen Klinikums. In R Lanz, editor, *Medizin und Management bei Katastrophen und Massenunfällen*, pages 101 – 104. Hans Huber, Bern, 1992.

[150] KD Kühn. Katastrophenvorsorge in Deutschland — Ein Jahr danach. *Bevölkerungsschutz — Magazin für Zivil- und Katastrophenschutz*, (4):47, 2002.

[151] W Künzi. Versorgung von Verbrennungsopfern im Hospitalisationsraum Europa. In *Symposium: Professionalität in besonderen Lagen*, Chur, 2/3 April 1998. Interverband für das Rettungswesen.

[152] Landesärztekammer Baden-Württemberg. Satzung der Landesärztekammer Baden-Württemberg über die Eignungsvoraussetzungen für Leitende Notärzte im Rettungsdienst vom 2. August 1995, 1995.

[153] Landtag Rheinland-Pfalz. Plenarprotokoll 11/32 – 11. Wahlperiode, 32. Sitzung, Mainz, Deutschhaus, Donnerstag, 8. September 1988.

[154] R Lange. Technische Einsatzleitung im Landkreis Hannover. In Mitschke [185], chapter 5.6, pages 246 – 249.

[155] M Liberman, D Mulder, and J Sampalis. Advanced or basic life support for trauma: meta-analysis and critical review of the literature. *J Trauma*, 49(4):584 – 599, Oct 2000.

[156] N Lindner and T Jäger. Feuer, Hochwasser, Unfälle und KIT: Malteser-SEG Sandkrug. *SEG – Zeitschrift für Schnell-Einsatz-Gruppen und erweiterten Rettungsdienst*, 7(6):246 – 248, 2000.

[157] A Linhardt. *Feuerwehr im Luftschutz 1926–1945*. Number 19 in Deutsche Brandschutzgeschichte. vfdb, Braunschweig, 2002.

[158] C Lippay. Bombenanschlag auf das World Trade Center. *SEG – Magazin für Schnelleinsatzgruppen*, 3(1):37 – 39, 1996.

[159] C Lippay. Positionsbestimmung im Nordosten: SEG zwischen RD und KatS. *SEG – Zeitschrift für Schnell-Einsatz-Gruppen und erweiterten Rettungsdienst*, 5(6):281 – 282, 1998.

[160] D Lockey, G Davies, and T Coats. Survival of trauma patients who have prehospital tracheal intubation without anaesthesia or muscle relaxants: observational study. *Br Med J*, 323:141, 21 July 2001.

[161] G Lohre and T Eisenreich. Die SEG der Johanniter in Köln. *SEG – Magazin für Schnelleinsatzgruppen*, 1(5):216 – 218, 1994.

[162] WT Longstreth, LA Cobb, CE Fahrenbruch, and MK Copass. Does age affect outcomes of out-of-hospital cardiopulmonary resuscitation? *JAMA*, 264(16):2109 – 2110, Oct 24–31 1990.

[163] J Luckhardt. Die Sonder-Einsatz-Gruppe Rettungsdienst der Feuerwehr Wuppertal. In Mitschke and Peter [187], chapter 11.4, pages 307 – 314.

[164] B Lutomsky and F Flake. Schnelle Hilfe von nebenan. First-Responder-Systeme: zwei Beispiele aus Niedersachsen und Bayern. *Rettungs-Magazin*, 1(2):82 – 85, März/April 1996.

[165] J Luxem. Jahresbericht 1999 der Leitenden Notarztgruppe Aschaffenburg: 20 Großschadenereignisse. *SEG – Zeitschrift für Schnell-Einsatz-Gruppen und erweiterten Rettungsdienst*, 7(4):234, 2000.

[166] J Maaß. Leitender Notarzt und Sonder-Einsatz-Gruppen: Der neue Weg im Katasrophenschutz? *Feuerwehr-Magazin*, 9(8):84 – 90, 1992.

[167] J Maaß. Berufsfeuerwehr München. Erste Hilfe bei vielen Verletzten. *SEG – Magazin für Schnelleinsatzgruppen*, 1(4):149 – 152, 1994.

[168] J Maaß. Rettung und Katastrophe. Zukunftsprojekt für Sanitätszüge in NRW. *SEG – Magazin für Schnelleinsatzgruppen*, 1(2):75 – 77, 1994.

[169] J Maaß. Die neue Einsatzeinheit (EE) im DRK. *SEG – Magazin für Schnelleinsatzgruppen*, 2(3):156 – 158, 1995.

[170] J Maaß. Abgerutscht. Busunglück in Winterberg/Hochsauerlandkreis (NRW). *Rettungs-Magazin*, 1(5):30 – 36, 1996.

[171] J Maaß. Rettungsdienst in Dortmund. Auf gute Nachbarschaft. *Rettungs-Magazin*, 1(6):18 – 29, 1996.

[172] J Maaß. Qualm-Falle. Brand auf dem Düsseldorfer Flughafen. *Rettungs-Magazin*, 2(1):38 – 45, 1997.

[173] DP Mackie and HM Koning. Fate of mass burn casualties: implications for disaster planning. *Burns*, 16(3):203 – 206, 1990.

[174] N Mangold. Ramstein 28.08 1988. http://www.muehlenbiker.de/Ramstein/ramstein.html, accessed 16/08/2003 2003.

[175] TE Martin. The ramstein airshow disaster. *J Royal Army Med Corps*, 136:19 – 26, 1990.

[176] F Marx. Das Schweizer Patientenleitsystem. Eine europäische Alternative zur Verletztenanhängekarte. *SEG – Magazin für Schnelleinsatzgruppen*, 1(6):238 – 239, 1994.

[177] M Masellis, A Iaia, G Sferrazza, E Pirillo, N D'Arpa, P Cucchiara, M Sucameli, B Napoli, G Alessandro, and S Giarni. Fire disaster in a motorway tunnel. *Annals of Burns and Fire Disasters*, 10(4):241 – 245, December 1997.

[178] K Maurer. Transportkapazitäten im Rettungsdienst. In Hierholzer and Böhm [116], pages 42 – 51.

[179] K Maurer. Logistik bei einem Massenanfall von Verletzten: Abrollbehälter. *SEG – Magazin für Schnelleinsatzgruppen*, 4(5):194 – 197, 1997.

[180] K Maurer, A Lechleuthner, B Bouillon, R Blohmeyer, and H Troidl. Zwei Jahre OrgL-Ausbildung in NRW. *SEG – Zeitschrift für Schnell-Einsatz-Gruppen und erweiterten Rettungsdienst*, 8(1):42 – 45, 2001.

[181] T Mauz. "Einsatz für 31 Emil". Rettungsdienst in Hamburg. *Rettungs-Magazin*, 2(1):18 – 29, 1997.

[182] G Maxisch. Das Zugunglück von Northeim. In Mitschke and Peter [187], chapter 12.2, pages 353 – 359.

[183] WMP McCall. *The American Ambulance 1900-2002*. Iconografix, Hudson, WI, 2002.

[184] T Mitschke. Einbindung der Schnell-Einsatz-Gruppen in die Führungsorganisation der Gefahrenabwehr. In Mitschke and Peter [187], chapter 7, pages 199 – 231.

[185] T Mitschke, editor. *Handbuch für Technische Einsatzleitungen*. Kohlhammer, Stuutgart, 1997.

[186] T Mitschke, J Kardel, and D Dietrich. *Einrichten und Betreiben von Bereitstellungsräumen*, volume 4 of *SEGmente*. Stumpf & Kossendey, Edewecht, 2002.

[187] T Mitschke and H Peter, editors. *Handbuch für Schnell-Einsatz-Gruppen*. Stumpf & Kossendey, Edewecht, 2nd edition, 1994.

[188] KH Muncke. Organisationspläne und Stärkenachweisungen von LS-Einheiten. In Koczy [148], pages 153 – 178.

[189] G Neff. Organisatorischer Leiter und Leitender Notarzt. In Crespin and Peter [65], chapter 3, pages 71 – 92.

[190] G Neff. Die Sichtung. In Crespin and Neff [64], chapter 2, pages 71 – 109.

[191] S Neuhauser. Versorgung eingeklemmter Patienten — Fallbeispiele. In Engelhardt [83], pages 474 – 477.

[192] R Noto, P Huguenard, and A Larcan. *Manual de medicina de catástrofe.* Masson, Barcelona, 1989.

[193] R Obladen and HP Milz. Dokumentationssystem für den MANV: Das Bielefelder System. *SEG – Magazin für Schnelleinsatzgruppen*, 6(2):62 – 17, 1999.

[194] Federal Minister of the Interior. Civil Defence in the Federal Republic of Germany. Bonn, 1980.

[195] SP O'Hickey, CA Pickering, PE Jones, and JD Evans. Manchester air disaster. *Br Med J*, 294(6588):1663 – 1667, 27 Jun 1987.

[196] S Osche. Neu, zweckmäßig, schnell und schön: Der neue KTW des Bundes. *Im Einsatz. Zeitschrift für Helfer und Führungskräfte*, 8:26 – 27, Oktober 2001.

[197] S Osche and F Zeiler. Die Anhängekarte für Verletzte/Kranke. In Crespin and Neff [64], chapter 3.5.4, pages 201 – 207.

[198] H Peter. Aufbau von SEG'en. *SEG – Magazin für Schnelleinsatzgruppen*, 1(4):147 – 148, 1994.

[199] H Peter. Voraussetzungen und Notwendigkeiten für den Aufbau von Schnelleinsatzgruppen. In Mitschke and Peter [187], chapter 1, pages 21 – 46.

[200] H Peter. Einsatzplanung. In Crespin and Peter [65], chapter 8, pages 155 – 174.

[201] H Peter. Einsatztaktik beim Massenanfall Verletzter: Ordnung des Raumes. *SEG – Magazin für Schnelleinsatzgruppen*, 4(4):150 – 153, 1997.

[202] H Peter. Eschede — Bilanz eines Einsatzes. *SEG – Magazin für Schnelleinsatzgruppen*, 5(4):170 – 172, 1998.

[203] H Peter. Neue MANV-Richtlinie in Bayern. *SEG – Zeitschrift für Schnell-Einsatz-Gruppen und erweiterten Rettungsdienst*, 7(1):31 – 32, 2000.

[204] H Peter and K Maurer, editors. *Die Leitstelle beim MANV.* Praxiswissen. Stumpf & Kossendey, Edewecht, 2001.

[205] H Peter and T Mitschke. Die neue Dienstvorschrift 100: Führung und Leitung im Einsatz. *Im Einsatz*, 8(4):28 – 29, 2001.

[206] H Peter, T Mitschke, and T Uhr. *Notarzt und Rettungsassistent beim MANV.* Number 3 in SEGmente. Stumpf & Kossendey, Edewecht, 1998.

[207] H Peter and JW Weidringer. *Der Verbandplatz.* Number 2 in SEGmente. Stumpf & Kossendey, Edewecht, 1998.

[208] H Peter and JW Weidringer. *Der Behandlungsplatz.* Number 2 in SEGmente. Stumpf & Kossendey, Edewecht, 2nd edition, 2001.

[209] S Peters. Forderungen des LNA an die Ausbildung der SEG für den MANV-Einsatz. *SEG – Magazin für Schnelleinsatzgruppen*, 2(3):124 – 125, 1995.

[210] E Pfenninger and D Hauber. *Medizinische Versorgung beim Massenanfall Verletzter bei Chemikalienfreisetzung.* Number 44 in Schriftenreihe der Schutzkommission beim Bundesminister des Inneren, Neue Folge. Bundesverwaltungsamt — Zentralstelle für Zivilschutz, Bonn, 2001.

[211] WJ Phillips, PC Reynolds, M Lenczyk, S Walton, and S Ciresi. Anesthesia during a mass-casualty disaster: The army's experience at fort bragg, north carolina, march 23, 1994. *Mil Med*, 162(6):371 – 373, June 1997.

[212] HP Plattner. Die Einsatzleitung in der Führungsorganisation zur zivilen Gefahrenabwehr. In Mitschke [185], chapter 2, pages 93 – 134.

[213] GM Pomerantz. *Nine Minutes Twenty Seconds.* Penguin Non-fiction. Penguin, London, 2003.

[214] E Preuß. *Eschede, 10 Uhr 59.* GeraMond, Munich, 1998.

[215] E Rebentisch. Geschichte der Sichtung. In Crespin and Neff [64], chapter 1.1, pages 31 – 40.

[216] R Rebmann. Busunfall an der A3. *SEG – Zeitschrift für Schnell-Einsatz-Gruppen und erweiterten Rettungsdienst*, 6(3):108, 1999.

[217] F Richter, B Tabuteau, E Cheftel, and A Michel. Attentat auf das regionale Schnellbahnnetz (RER) bei der Station Saint-Michel. *SEG – Magazin für Schnelleinsatzgruppen*, 3(1):40 – 42, 1996.

[218] KH Rosen. Reform im Zivil- und Katastrophenschutz. Grußwort des Abteilungsleiters O im Bundesministerium des Inneren auf der 51. Sitzung der Schutzkommission beim BMI am 9./10. Mai 2002 in Trier, http://www.bzsbund.de/rede_rosen_sk.pdf, 2002.

[219] JM Rowles and DC Bouch. The injuries sustained in the m1 plane crash. In Wallace et al. [261], chapter 3, pages 29 – 46.

[220] JR Saffle. The 1942 fire at boston's cocoanut grove nightclub. *Am J Surg*, 166:581 – 591, December 1993.

[221] A Sauaia, FA Moore, EE Moore, KS Moser, R Brennan, RA Read, and PT Pons. Epidemiology of trauma deaths: A reassessment. *J Trauma*, 38(2):185 – 193, 1998.

[222] K Schlitz. Schnell–Einsatz–Gruppe Wangen. *SEG – Magazin für Schnelleinsatzgruppen*, 1(3):124 – 125, 1994.

[223] U Schmidt, SB Frame, ML Nerlich, DW Rowe, BL Enderson, KI Maull, and H Tscherne. On-scene helicopter transport of patients with multiple injuries–comparison of a german and an american system. *J Trauma*, 33(4):548 – 555, Oct 1992.

[224] DU Schmidt-Herholz. Großunfall. *Feuerwehr-Magazin*, 9(3):34 – 48, 1992.

[225] R Schmitt. Schnell-Einsatz-Gruppe Heilbronn 2: Eine engagierte SEG mit "Chemie-Know-How". *SEG – Magazin für Schnelleinsatzgruppen*, 3(6):390 – 391, 1996.

[226] L Schmitz-Eggen. 18. Januar 1996. Die Brandnacht von Lübeck. *Rettungs-Magazin*, 1(4):30 – 35, 1996.

[227] L Schmitz-Eggen. Das ICE Unglück von Eschede. *Rettungs-Magazin*, 4(5):30 – 35, 1998.

[228] L Schmitz-Eggen. EXPO. Solo für die Feuerwehr. *Rettungs-Magazin*, 5(5):66 – 75, 2000.

[229] L Schmitz-Eggen. Grenzenlose Hilfe. *Rettungs-Magazin*, 5(5):23 – 26, 2000.

[230] L Schmitz-Eggen. Nächtliche Entgleisung. *Rettungs-Magazin*, 5:36 – 42, 2000.

[231] L Schmitz-Eggen. 80 Stunden im Einsatz. *Rettungs-Magazin*, 6(3):66 – 71, 2001.

[232] L Schmitz-Eggen. Fataler Kunstfehler: Das Flugschau-Unglück in Ramstein. *Rettungs-Magazin*, 6(4):85, 2001.

[233] L Schmitz-Eggen. Schock fürs Leben. Frühdefibrillation durch Laien. *Rettungs-Magazin*, 6(4):30 – 34, 2001.

[234] L Schmitz-Eggen. Tödlicher Ausflug. *Rettungs-Magazin*, 6(5):44, 2001.

[235] L Schmitz-Eggen and J Maaß. Herborn in Flammen. *Rettungs-Magazin*, 5(4):59, 2000.

[236] M Schneider. Betr. Busunglück mit SEG-Einsatz. *SEG – Magazin für Schnelleinsatzgruppen*, 1(2):82, 1994.

[237] T Schneider. Frühdefibrillationsprogramm Mainz/Multicenterstudie. *alert*, (2):30 – 32, 1994.

[238] H Scholl and E Nagel. Memorandum für europaweite Luftrettung. *Rettungsdienst*, 20:1045 – 1047, 11 1997.

[239] M Schrömbgens. Gesetz zur Neuordnung des Zivilschutzes. Seine Auswirkungen auf die Hilfsorganisationen und deren Mitarbeiter. *SEG – Magazin für Schnelleinsatzgruppen*, 4(3):118 – 120, 1997.

[240] Schutzkommission beim Bundesminister des Innern, editor. *Katastrophenmedizin. Leitfaden für die ärztliche Versorgung im Katastrophenfall.* Der Bundesminister des Innern, Bonn, 1981.

[241] P Sefrin. Massenanfall von Verletzten und Erkrankten in der modernen Industriegesellschaft. Betrachtungen zu einem aktuellen Thema. *Bevölkerungsschutz — Magazin für Zivil- und Katastrophenschutz*, (3):3 – 7, 1998.

[242] W Sladek. Der neue Großraumrettungswagen (Rettungsbus) der Berufsfeuerwehr Köln. *SEG – Magazin für Schnelleinsatzgruppen*, 1(5):186 – 188, 1994.

[243] G Smith. Special report: Big explosion in a small town. *National Fire & Rescue*, 27(2):10 – 13, March/April 2003.

[244] Ständige Konferenz für Katastrophenvorsorge und Katastrophenschutz (SKK). Dienstvorschrift 100, Führung und Leitung im Einsatz, 1999.

[245] T Standl, E Cavus, and HR Paschen. Der Einfluß der Frühdefibrillation auf die Überlebensrate nach CPR im Rettungsdienst der Stadt Hamburg. In Engelhardt [83], pages 370 – 373.

[246] TM Stein. Mass shootings. In DE Hogan and JL Burstein, editors, *Disaster Medicine*, chapter 36, pages 376 – 384. Lippincott Williams & Wilkins, Philadelphia, 2002.

[247] IH Stevens and R Partridge. The clapham rail disaster. *Injury*, 21:37 – 40, 1990.

[248] U Stiaßny. Gasexplosion in Wohnhausanlage. Einsatzbericht aus Niederösterreich. *SEG – Zeitschrift für Schnell-Einsatz-Gruppen und erweiterten Rettungsdienst*, 7(1):11 – 13, 2000.

[249] D Stratmann. Aufgaben des 'Leitenden Notarztes'. In Hierholzer and Böhm [116], pages 1 – 6

[250] P Tatlow. *Harrow & Wealdstone 50 Years on. Clearing up the Aftermath.* X75. Oakwood Press, Usk, 2002.

[251] K Thäsler. Aspekte aus der Sicht der Medien. In Hüls and Oestern [127], chapter 5.3, pages 147 – 149.

[252] DD Trunkey. Trauma. *Scientific American*, 249(2):20 –27, August 1983.

[253] A Trupka, C Waydhas, D Nast-Kolb, and L Schweiberer. Early intubation in severely injured patients. *Eur J Emerg Med*, 1(1):1 – 8, Mar 1994.

[254] K Tucker and A Lettin. The tower of london bomb explosion. *Br Med J*, 3:287 – 289, 2 August 1975.

[255] T Uhr. Maßnahmen des ersteintreffenden Rettungsteams beim Rettungsdienst Einsatz mit Massenanfall Betroffener. In Engelhardt [82], pages 275 – 279.

[256] T Uhr. Sichtungsstrategien und Sichtungsverfahren ersteintreffender Rettungskräfte. In Crespin and Neff [64], chapter 3.1, pages 110 – 117.

[257] T Vemmer. Großveranstaltungen: Ein Blick über den Ärmelkanal. *SEG – Zeitschrift für Schnell-Einsatz-Gruppen und erweiterten Rettungsdienst*, 6(3):123 – 124, 1999.

[258] S Volz. Intensiv-Transport-Hubschrauber. Die Klinik-Hüpfer. *Rettungs-Magazin*, 2(4):32 – 36, 1997.

[259] S Volz. Johanniter auf Bergtour. *Rettungs-Magazin*, 6(1):70 – 74, 2001.

[260] S Volz. Starker Rücken. *Rettungs-Magazin*, 6(4):18 – 29, 2001.

[261] WA Wallace, JM Rowles, and CL Colton, editors. *Management of disasters and their aftermath.* BMJ Publishing Group, London, 1994.

[262] J Wardrope. Crush asphyxia and management of "unannounced" major incidents, with experiences from hillsborough. In Wallace et al. [261], chapter 16, pages 235 – 247.

[263] TA Waterworth and MJT Carr. Report on injuries sustained by patients treated at the birmingham general hospital following the recent bomb explosions. *Br Med J*, 2:25 – 27, 5 April 1975.

[264] JW Weidringer, J Leichtle, and R Stern, editors. *Großunfall Symposium '89. Interdisziplinäre Überlegungen und Einsatzberichte.* ASB Arbeiter-Samariter-Bund Landesverband Bayern, Ortsverband Illertissen, München, 1990. Werner Wolfsfellner Medizinverlag.

[265] B Wetzenbacher. Verbandplatz Bahnhofshalle. Zugunglück von Garmisch-Partenkirchen (Bayern). *Rettungs-Magazin*, 1(2):32 – 37, März/April 1996.

[266] B Wetzenbacher. Die Stunde der Flieger. Gelenkbus umgestürzt — 29 Verletzte auf der Autobahn A7 bei Neu-Ulm (Bayern). *Rettungs-Magazin*, 3(1):57 – 60, 1998.

[267] JP Wilke. Zwischen allen Fronten. In JP Wilke, editor, *150 Jahre Berliner Feuerwehr. 1851 – 2001*, pages 78 – 83. FKF Media, Berlin, 2001.

[268] KP Wresch. Flugzeugabsturz in Ramstein: Erfahrungen bei der rettungsdienstlichen Bewältigung des Großunfalls. In Weidringer et al. [264], pages 62 – 68.

[269] Gesetz zur Neuordnung des Zivilschutzes. Bundesgesetzblatt 1, 726ff, 1997.